SHAMBHALA DRAGON EDITIONS

The dragon is an age-old symbol of the highest spiritual essence, embodying wisdom, strength, and the divine power of transformation. In this spirit, Shambhala Dragon Editions offers a treasury of readings in the sacred knowledge of Asia. In presenting the works of authors both ancient and modern, we seek to make these teachings accessible to lovers of wisdom everywhere.

LIVING
at the SOURCE

Yoga Teachings of
Vivekananda

Edited by
ANN MYREN &
DOROTHY MADISON

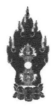

SHAMBHALA
Boston & London
1993

Shambhala Publications, Inc.
Horticultural Hall
300 Massachusetts Avenue
Boston, Massachusetts 02115
www.shambhala.com

Printed in the United States of America
Distributed in the United States by Random House, Inc.,
and in Canada by Random House of Canada Ltd

LIBRARY OF CONGRESS CATALOGING-IN-PUBLICATION DATA

Vivekananda, Swami, 1863–1902.
    [Complete works of Swami Vivekananda. Selections]
    Living at the source: Yoga teachings of Vivekananda /
    edited by Ann Myren and Dorothy Madison.—1st ed.
        p.   cm.—(Shambhala dragon editions)
    Selections from: The complete works of Swami Vivekananda. Cf. Pref.
    ISBN 1-57062-616-2 (pbk.)
    1. Spiritual life—Hinduism.   2. Hinduism—Doctrines.
    3. Ramakrishna Mission.   I. Myren, Ann.   II. Madison, Dorothy.
    III. Title.
BL1280.292.V58A25   1993   92-56450
294.5'4—dc20   CIP
    BVG 01

This book is for Vivekananda's "other God"—you, and the whole of humankind.

Everything in the universe is struggling to complete a circle, to return to its source, to return to its only real Source, the Self.

—VIVEKANANDA

This is the Lord of all, the Knower of all, the Inner Controller. This is the Source of all, the beginning and end of all beings.

—MANDUKYA UPANISHAD

CONTENTS

CONTENTS

PREFACE

VIVEKANANDA appeared on the American scene at the Parliament of Religions during the World's Columbian Exhibition in Chicago in 1893. In his very first speech, he began with the words "Sisters and Brothers of America." This warm and sincere greeting, addressed to an audience of several thousand, stirred his listeners who responded with an ovation of several minutes. Here was a man with a message of tolerance, a plea to end bigotry, an appeal to recognize the equal truth of all religions, and an assertion of the innate divinity of every man, woman, and child. It was a new message for America. Such affinity developed between Vivekananda and Americans that he stayed in the West from 1893 to 1897, and came a second time from 1899 to 1900, teaching to one and all.

We have compiled this book of Vivekananda's teachings, *Living at the Source*, in order to commemorate his appearance at the Parliament of Religions, and to make known his contribution to the living stream of spirituality in America. It is in keeping with Vivekananda's embrace of the whole of America that some fifty Vedantins from all parts of the country worked on the material for *Living at the Source*. This group not only selected Vivekananda's words from the eight volumes of *The Complete Works of Swami Vivekananda*, but many of them also participated in other tasks in the preparation of this book.

In view of the fact that the quest for self-knowledge has so many different starting points, the chapters of *Living at the Source* do not follow any particular order. The reader could just as well begin with "The Human Condition" as with "Who Am I?," "Work as Self-Transformation," or any other chapter that captures his or her interest. Indeed, to readers who prefer to think independently, a set chapter order may not be at all appealing. Rather, they may want to browse through *Living at the Source* to discover for themselves their own way to self-knowledge. In any case, it is possible to form a practical philosophy based on these selections from Vivekananda's works.

We want to call attention to two matters. First, Vivekananda wrote and spoke in the language of his times. Consequently, he used the words *man, men,* and *mankind* to refer to women as well as men. It was never his intention to favor one gender over the other. And second, in the subtitle, *The Yoga Teachings of Vivekananda,* we have used the word *yoga* to describe his teachings. "Yoga" means union of the personal self with God, or the universal Self. Vivekananda himself used *yoga* to describe his teachings when he first taught in America. Later he called his teachings "Vedanta."

The selections that follow are taken from Vivekananda's lectures, class talks, letters, newspaper interviews, and conversations. Each selection is followed by a volume and page citation indicating where it appears in the *Complete Works of Swami Vivekananda* (paper, 1984–87).

ACKNOWLEDGMENTS

THE VIVEKANANDA FOUNDATION wishes to acknowledge the assistance of all those who participated in the compilation of *Living at the Source*. Mel Margolis, whose self-chosen title, "working stiff," truly describes him, and text preparation expert Diana Lorentz were especially helpful in moving the project along without hitches or setbacks. We also want to thank Kendra Crossen, managing editor of Shambhala Publications, for her editorial skill as well as her patience, kindness, and consideration.

We are grateful to all the Vedantins who generously gave their time to the selection of excerpts from Vivekananda's works. This group includes the following lay persons and monastics: Richard Allen, Swami Atmarupananda, Swami Atmavartananda, Ray Berry, Swami Bhaveshananda, Uli Burgin, Nirvana Chaitanya, William E. Corcoran, Mary G. Corson, John Dobson, Violet A. Eaton, Kathleen Giustino, Gail T. Gregory, Erik Johns, Cliff Johnson, Thelma and Jack Lindow, Sandy K. Martin, Marilyn McIver, Kumar Mehta, Margie Miles, Martha Muirhead, Nachiketa, Mira Nenonen, Alex Pappas, Sandra Winkler Rajan, Swami Sahajananda, Pravrajika Sarvatmaprana, Edwin Schroeder, Steven F. Walker, Dennis Yniguez, and Frederick A. Zulch. Our thanks also to those who prefer to remain unnamed.

A great share of the selecting and editing was done by the assistant editors: Brahmacharini Ishani, Ann Kenny, Carolyn Kenny, Leta Jane Lewis, George Rigby, Nell Siena, Pravrajika Vrajaprana, and Swami Yogeshananda, all of whom gave unstintingly of their time, intelligence, perceptiveness, analytical abilities, and good-heartedness.

We also want to thank Swami Asitananda, who was especially helpful with proofreading; Ted Chenoweth, who helped with mailing lists; and the Vedanta Society of Southern California, for permission to use several selections that first appeared in *Vedanta and the West* and were later included in *The Complete Works of Swami Vivekananda*.

INTRODUCTION

*L*IVING AT THE SOURCE is powerful medicine. Like remedies straight from God and Nature, the ideas and utterances in this book act directly on life, mind, and spirit. Their tenor is strength, because "strength is the medicine for the world's disease."[1] Geared to the facts of the workaday world, yet powerfully attuned to the true and the holy, they strike a supremely human nerve. Stirring the will, they set in motion all kinds of strivings for self-knowledge, spiritual wholeness, generosity of spirit, and "courage never to submit or yield." All the sting, salt, and savor of prophetic discourse stamp this book; it lives, makes live, and cuts through delusion.

The prophet whose words and ideas animate *Living at the Source* is the great Indian monk Swami Vivekananda. A century ago Americans hailed him as the man of the hour, but now his name is rarely heard. When he landed in America in 1893, Vivekananda was thirty years old, fit and daring—a do-or-die hero tempered in fire and holiness. He had a labor to perform. His dying master, Shri Ramakrishna, had written on a scrap of paper: "Naren [Vivekananda] will teach people when he will speak with a raised voice at home and outside."[2] And so it happened. America was the land where he first raised his voice, and where he forged his message. "I call upon men," he said, "to make themselves conscious of their divinity within."[3] To understand this holy stranger, his quality and force—indeed, to have any idea of Vivekananda at all—we begin with the facts of his life. These, as out-of-the-ordinary as they are, can be ticked off quickly; the challenge is to make sense of them and grasp their significance. What we relate here is the merest run-through, but necessary for all that.

Vivekananda was born in India, then a British colony administered by the East India Company; the date was 12 January 1863, a few days after Lincoln had signed the Emancipation Proclamation. Vivekananda's family, the aristocratic Dattas of Calcutta, named him, their first surviving son, Narendranath. He throve, acted, and came to manhood with a bearing not unlike that of a Renaissance prince. It was a manner he kept even as a monk wandering India's hills and heartlands.

As a child Narendranath was quick, audacious, and alive to his fingertips. Headstrong and not to be interfered with, he led first his mother, then others, on a merry chase. But because he was handsome and talented and provided wonderful company, friends crowded around him. In school and college he was in constant demand. There was no reason at all why he should not have enjoyed his enchanted life to the full. And so he did, until the time came when his fastidious Indian intellect seized upon the theories and practices of the Western life and mind. Attracted and easily subverted, first by the West's readiness to reason its way to truth and beauty, and second, by its active, often bloody quest for liberty and social justice, Narendranath began to acquire his unusual mastery of the West's history and intellectual tradition. Indeed, his early identification with the mind of the West remained lifelong.

Meanwhile, into the midst of his intellectual joy crashed unreason's thunderbolt. This was God, Whom Narendranath had always loved and meditated upon, but Whom reason could not prove to exist. So now, driven not only by the love of learning, but by the desire for God, he searched for a genuine God-authority. He became a kind of roving threat, asking first this holy man and then that one his forthright question: "Sir, have you seen God?"

At last, Shri Ramakrishna Paramahamsa, who dwelled in a temple-garden outside Calcutta, answered him a vigorous yes, and played his bold questioner like a fish. Narendranath had met his Master. He also found God during a six-year period filled with spiritual incident and human woe. After initial revolts and continuing protests against his Master's counsel—mainly in the name of reason—he experienced God in His many states and aspects, and realized his own eternal oneness with the divine Self. On the human side, his father's sudden death hurled Narendranath's family to the edge of ruin, and himself into the job market. As if that were not enough, Ramakrishna died two years later, leaving him in charge of a dozen brother-disciples, all of them spiritual giants, eager to renounce the world for a life in God.

During the next years, from 1887 to 1893, Narendranath lived either with his brother monks in their makeshift monastery or by himself on the open road. His experience as a wandering monk all but undid him. Although his own holy-man hardships toughened his fiber and tempered his steel, the cradle-to-grave hardships of India's people sent him into bouts of grief and despair that precipitated a chronic anguish. The direct encounter with India's broken, impoverished people transformed him once and for all; every last drop of elitism was drained out of him, every concern for himself dissolved. His only recourse was to devise a plan to raise up his people, the wretched of the earth. In this wise, and with this end in view, he came to America.

The occasion seemed ready-made: that year, 1893, Chicago's great Columbian Exposition was to include a Parliament of Religions, to which representatives of all the world religions had been invited. It was to this parliament that Narendranath, now known as Vivekananda, came unknown and uninvited. A handful of enthusiastic friends and disciples, mainly from Madras, outfitted him and paid for his passage.

At the Parliament Vivekananda raised his voice high and found himself famous. Many reasons have been advanced for his instant acclaim: the substance and energy of his talks, the magnetism of his presence, the youth and beauty of his person, the magic of his eloquence, his fierce sincerity and bursts of humor, the range and power of his intellect. To the popular mind he was glamour to feast on; to the cultivated mind, a shock never fully sustained.

Vivekananda was fully aware of the stir he was causing, but he was not diverted from trying to raise money for India. His idea was to send the proceeds from his lectures around the country to his brother monks and disciples in India; they, in turn, would equip themselves to go out among India's villages, bringing men, women, and children the rudiments of knowledge. Education, not religion, was his first prescription for raising up his people.

This plan never succeeded. The reasons for Vivekananda's failure to earn enough, and the tremendous work he did accomplish in India notwithstanding, can be passed over. For Americans, the critical fact is that during this first Western sojourn of roughly three years, Vivekananda immersed himself in the American ethos so thoroughly that he became American in spirit and in a certain sense America's prophet. With raised voice and plain words he made clear to the American people their inmost identity, the Self; and he exhorted them to shake off the hypnotic inertia hiding this infinite Divinity within. Inevitably, out of the argument, energy, and direction of his reasoning, Vivekananda gave new life and meaning to the self-evident truths upon which America stood. In essence, he told Americans that they could not have the one without the other: they could not experience themselves as the Self, without the perfect practice of freedom and equality. Nor could they have perfect freedom and equality without knowledge of the Self.

Yet Vivekananda's swift synthesis of his own spiritual humanism with America's democratic ideals was not deliberate. It simply happened, like a chemical reaction. Here was a Hindu holy man to whom, quite literally, nothing human was alien; and around him buzzed and crackled this new, confident, tremendously open and vital society, with whom he rubbed elbows. In no time at all he loved this "Yankee land" and became as Yankee as the next. Yet he remained spiritual to the core. He was, in sum, a new type of man, the prototype of a new ideal—the spiritual democrat.

Inevitably, the "Americanization" of Vivekananda developed a terrific spiritual spin because of his master-reflex to spiritualize everything. In plain English, he perceived as divine the whole of reality, including the traits, values, and practices of human society. Further, he was able to see at once which "American" ideas, attitudes, and practices contributed to human wholeness and spiritual well-being, and which of these traits were indispensable. These came to figure in his message to the world-at-large and have become inextricably united with the spiritual aims and methods of "Practical Vedanta."

Vedanta is the philosophy of the Upanishads, India's ancient sacred texts; it is also the bedrock upon which India's diverse theologies and religions rest. Because the seed-concept of Vivekananda's message—the identity of the individual soul with the universal soul—came straight out of the Upanishads, he called his message "Vedanta." And it was "practical," because he wanted all men and women to live in the conscious grip of this truth—as, indeed, he himself did—and as he believed Americans were ready to do. In his view, the particular American attitudes and behaviors that enabled them to get on in life also fitted them for the pursuit of Self-knowledge.

Especially did the Americans' faith in themselves stir Vivekananda; it was part of that brisk cluster of strengths he associated with Self-knowledge. He perceived this excellent strength in their love of independence, in the ways they figured things out for themselves, stood up for themselves, and looked after themselves, welcoming the new and taking setbacks in stride. It also showed in the way they worked, using every kind of skill in the book and inventing others along the way. And he admired their penchant for heading into the future, all heart, sinew, and sweat. They did not wait for things to happen or for God to make their decisions for them; instead, they saluted reason, used common sense, took their chances and went ahead, propelled by no one but themselves.

This voltage of pluck and enterprise struck Vivekananda the day he set foot on Chicago's fairgrounds. His real vetting probably began when he noticed the female presence. Unlike the secluded women of India, American women were everywhere, self-directed and fearless. The spacious, object-filled Woman's Building, designed and managed by women themselves, shouted to high heaven of freedom and equality. The men, no less than the women, responded to freedom's cry. Even the low and beggarly demanded and got respect; no law, custom, or caste could block their upward climb.

These various traits, which had so taken Vivekananda by storm, never ceased to inspire him. They mirrored his own traits, of course, but in America he kept witnessing them en masse under multiple working conditions—effortlessly acted out, so to speak, on a nationwide scale. It was little wonder that he sometimes sounded American himself. In India he said, "Liberty is the first condition of growth."[4] In Oakland: "I have never seen a man who was not at least my equal."[5] In Chicago he was quoted as saying, "The idea of perfect womanhood is perfect independence"[6] and in Detroit he said: "The salvation of your country depends upon its women."[7] In San Francisco: "If it is strength, go down into hell and get hold of it."[8] And he continued in this vein in India, ending a lecture there by saying:

> All power is within you; you can do anything and everything. Believe in that, do not believe that you are weak; do not believe that you are half-crazy lunatics, as most of us do nowadays. You can do anything and everything without even the guidance of anyone. All power is there. Stand up and express the divinity within you.[9]

But no matter how open, forthright, and congenial they were, America's strengths did not conceal from Vivekananda's eye the "dollar-worship" that gripped the men or the sensation-seeking that diminished the women. These and other blots on American conduct and character he did not hesitate to haul over the coals. Nevertheless, he believed that Americans still had a chance to become the balanced, powerful, spiritual people the world so badly needed: they were democrats.

Vivekananda recommended no set religious beliefs for these new people. He wanted them to practice a religion of their own choosing (for all paths lead to God) or even to invent one to suit themselves. The fact is that he loved the diversity of paths just as he loved the diversity of people who traveled them. From this one simple fact stemmed the many ways he talked about the relationship between God, soul, and nature. His subject matter ranged from the formless Absolute to God the Father, the Mother, and the Divine Child. He spoke of seeking God within our heart, of perceiving God as the external universe, and of worshiping God as "the other God—man." Again, he urged that when in doubt we follow our heart; but he also urged that we follow reason, analyzing our way to impersonal Truth. Indeed, Vivekananda's teachings abound in every kind of metaphor, attitude, argument, and principle. But every one of them without exception is valid from a given standpoint, reference, or circumstance.

At root level, however, underlying both religious particulars and questions of temperament, Vivekananda wanted every human being to "stand on the Self." "Stand as a rock," he said. "You are indestructible. You are the Self, the God of the universe."[10] His position in this matter is crystal clear. By affirming one's identity with the Self—with one's own inborn, boundless, and profoundly intimate divinity—all one's strengths become intensified and one's self-sense is transformed.

In Vivekananda's own experience, it was this sovereign unity of God, man, and universe that eclipsed all facts bearing upon the conduct of life, the knowledge of God, and the mastery of oneself. In no way does this unity impose limits on human thought or behavior; the more diversity, the better. For operating deep within the human psyche, unity expands, lifts, and unifies consciousness, so that objects, events, emotions, and life itself acquire new and richer meaning. Best of all—and most necessary—knowledge of this unity yanks out fear by the roots.

The infinite Self, with whom the liberated are indissolubly one although they live and move in the world of the many, is the source and fountainhead of pure joy. This is the joy that suffused Vivekananda's behavior and smoothed his edges, as he moved about performing his Master's labor. On visits to England in 1895 and 1896, he taught inspired by the same great joy and power he had conveyed in America. And on his return to India in 1897, he prescribed and dispensed to the people his joyous, powerful medicine, called by him the "Religion of Man-making."

Once again coming to the United States in 1899–1900, he gave in San Francisco what many regard as his highest, most extreme, least cushioned discourses. As he lashed into hypocrisy, heedlessness, self-love, and superstition, he scattered the terrible, stripped-down truths of the sages. The prophet in him was uppermost; he was thirty-seven and time was running out.

On 4 July 1902, a year and a half after he returned to India, Vivekananda died. Even now his legacy is not fully understood. But certain things are definite. He founded two American Vedanta Societies, one in New York, the other in San Francisco. In India he left behind a small, pure, extremely powerful monastic organization, with many programs to succor and raise the people. And to each of us—to humanity at large—he left straight, flinty speech about our common, innate divinity, and the ways and means for us to take possession of it.

NOTES

1. Swami Vivekananda, *The Complete Works of Swami Vivekananda*, Mayavati Memorial Edition, 8 vols. (Calcutta: Advaita Ashrama, 1984–1987), 2:201.
2. D. P. Gupta and D. K. Sengupta, eds., *Sri Sri Ramakrishna Kathamrita Centenary Memorial* (Chandigarh, India: Sri Ma Trust, 1982) p. 157.
3. *Complete Works*, 5:187–88.
4. Ibid., 3:246.
5. Ibid., 6:48.
6. Ibid., 8:198.
7. Ibid., 3:510.
8. Ibid., 1:479.
9. Ibid., 3:284.
10. Ibid., 2:236.

LIVING AT THE SOURCE

1

WHO AM I?

External Coverings

We see, then, that this human being is composed first of this external covering, the body; second, the finer body, consisting of mind, intellect, and egoism. Behind them is the real Self of man. We have seen that all the qualities and powers of the gross body are borrowed from the mind; and the mind, the finer body, borrows its powers and luminosity from the soul, standing behind. (2:216)

We believe that every being is divine, is God. Every soul is a sun covered over with clouds of ignorance; the difference between soul and soul is owing to the difference in density of these layers of clouds. (4:357)

We know neither the subconscious, nor the superconscious. We know the conscious only. If a man stands up and says, "I am a sinner," he makes an untrue statement because he does not know himself. He is the most ignorant of men; of himself he knows only one part, because his knowledge covers only a part of the ground he is on. (2:449)

The mistake is that we cling to the body when it is the spirit that is really immortal. (4:244)

He who says he is the body is a born idolater. We are spirit, spirit that has no form or shape, spirit that is infinite, and not matter. (2:40)

Some people are so afraid of losing their individuality. Wouldn't it be better for the pig to lose his pig-individuality if he can become God? Yes. But the poor pig does not think so at the time. Which state is my individuality? When I was a baby sprawling on the floor trying to swallow my thumb? Was that the individuality I should be sorry to lose? Fifty years hence I shall look upon this present state and laugh, just as I [now] look upon the baby state. Which of these individualities shall I keep? (2:467)

Mother, father, child, wife, body, wealth—everything I can lose except my Self . . . bliss in the Self. All desire is contained in the Self. . . . This is individuality which never changes, and this is perfect. (2:468)

This Very Soul Is the Self in All

In this external world, which is full of finite things, it is impossible to see and find the Infinite. The Infinite must be sought in that alone which is infinite, and the only thing infinite about us is that which is within us, our own soul. Neither the body, nor the mind, not even our thoughts, nor the world we see around us, are infinite. The Seer, He to whom they all belong, the Soul of man, He who is awake in the internal man, alone is infinite, and to seek for the Infinite Cause of this whole universe we must go there. In the Infinite Soul alone we can find it. (2:175)

The Soul is not composed of any materials. It is unity indivisible. Therefore it must be indestructible. For the same reasons it must also be without any beginning. So the Soul is without any beginning and end. (2:428)

There is no such thing as good and bad, they are not two different things; the same thing is good or bad, and the difference is only in degree. The very thing I call pleasurable today, tomorrow under better circumstances I may call pain. The fire that warms us can also consume us; it is not the fault of the fire. Thus, the Soul being

2

pure and perfect, the man who does evil is giving the lie unto himself, he does not know the nature of himself. Even in the murderer the pure Soul is there; It dies not. It was his mistake; he could not manifest It; he had covered It up. Nor in the man who thinks that he is killed is the Soul killed; It is eternal. (2:168)

After every happiness comes misery; they may be far apart or near. The more advanced the soul, the more quickly does one follow the other. *What we want is neither happiness nor misery.* Both make us forget our true nature; both are chains—one iron, one gold; behind both is the Atman, who knows neither happiness nor misery. These are *states*, and states must ever change; but the nature of the Soul is bliss, peace, unchanging. We have not to get it, we have it; only wash away the dross and see it.

Stand upon the Self, then only can we truly love the world. Take a very, very high stand; knowing our universal nature, we must look with perfect calmness upon all the *panorama* of the world. (7:11)

But as a man sees his own face in a mirror, perfect, distinct, and clear, so is the Truth shining in the soul of man. The highest heaven, therefore, is in our own souls; the greatest temple of worship is the human soul. (2:184)

The whole universe is one. There is only one Self in the universe, only One Existence, and that One Existence, when it passes through the forms of time, space, and causation, is called by different names, buddhi, fine matter, gross matter, all mental and physical forms. Everything in the universe is that One, appearing in various forms. When a little part of it comes, as it were, into this network of time, space, and causation it takes forms; take off the network, and it is all one. Therefore in the Advaita philosophy, the whole universe is all one in the Self which is called Brahman. That Self when it appears behind the universe is called God. The same Self when it appears behind this little universe, the body, is the soul. This very soul, therefore, is the Self in man. (2:461)

And in the midst of the depths of misery and degradation, the Soul sends a ray of light, and man wakes up and finds that what is really his, he can never lose. No, we can never lose what is really ours. Who can lose his being? Who can lose his every existence? If I am good, it is the existence first, and then that becomes colored with the quality of goodness. If I am evil, it is the existence first, and that becomes colored with the quality of badness. That existence is first, last, and always; it is never lost, but ever present.

Therefore, there is hope for all. None can die; none can be degraded forever. Life is but a playground, however gross the play may be. However we may receive blows, and however knocked about we may be, the Soul is there and is never injured. We are that Infinite. (2:402)

If I Am God

If I am God, I am beyond the tendencies of the senses and will not do evil. Morality, of course, is not the goal of man but the means through which this freedom is attained. (5:282)

You, as body, mind, or soul, are a dream, but what you really are, is Existence, Knowledge, Bliss. You are the God of this universe. You are creating the whole universe and drawing it in. (1:403)

All that is real in me is He; all that is real in Him is I. The gulf between God and man is thus bridged. Thus we find how, by knowing God, we find the kingdom of heaven within us. (1:323)

There is one thing to be remembered: that the assertion—I am God—cannot be made with regard to the sense-world. (5:282)

God is neither knowable nor unknowable, but something infinitely higher than either. He is one with us; and that which is one with us is neither knowable nor unknowable, as our own self. You cannot know your own self; you cannot move it out and make it an object to look at, because you *are* that and cannot separate yourself from it. Neither is it unknowable, for what is better known than yourself? It is really the center of our knowledge. In exactly the same sense, God is neither unknowable nor known, but infinitely higher than both; for He is our real Self. (2:134)

I have divided myself into God and me; I become the worshiped and I worship myself. Why not? God is I. Why not worship my Self? The universal God—He is also my Self. It is all fun. There is no other purpose. (2:471)

You Are Infinite

God is true. The universe is a dream. Blessed am I that I know this moment that I shall be free all eternity . . . that I know that I am worshiping only myself; that no nature, no delusion, had any hold on me. Vanish nature from me, vanish [these] gods; vanish worship . . . vanish superstitions, for I know myself. I am the Infinite. All these—Mrs. So-and-so, Mr. So-and-so, responsibility, happiness, misery—have vanished. I am the Infinite. How can there be death for me, or birth? Whom shall I fear? I am the One. Shall I be afraid of myself? Who is to be afraid of whom? I am the one Existence. Nothing else exists. I am everything. (1:501)

You are infinite. Where can you go? The sun, the moon, and the whole universe are but drops in your transcendent nature. How can you be born or die? I never was born, never will be born. I never had father or mother, friends or foes, for I am Existence, Knowledge, Bliss Absolute. (1:403)

Perfection is always infinite. We are this infinite already, and we are trying to manifest that infinity. You and I, and all beings, are trying to manifest it. (2:172)

The Bottom of the Lake

The bottom of a lake we cannot see, because its surface is covered with ripples. It is only possible for us to catch a glimpse of the bottom, when the ripples have subsided, and the water is calm. If the water is muddy or is agitated all the time, the bottom will not be seen. If it is clear, and there are no waves, we shall see the bottom. The bottom of the lake is our own true Self. (1:202)

You are the omniscient, omnipresent being of the universe. But of such beings can there be many? Can there be a hundred thousand million omnipresent beings? Certainly not. Then what becomes of us all? You are only one; there is only one such Self, and that One Self is you. (2:235)

While we recognize a God, it is really only the Self that we have separated from ourselves and worship as outside of us; but all the time it is our own true Self, the one and only God. (8:30)

The Self—the Atman—is by Its own nature pure. It is the same, the one Existence of the universe that is reflecting Itself from the lowest worm to the highest and most perfect being. The whole of this universe is one Unity, one Existence, physically, mentally, morally and spiritually. We are looking upon this one Existence in different forms and creating all these images upon It. (2:249)

Picture the Self to be the rider and this body the chariot, the intellect to be the charioteer, mind the reins, and the senses the horses. He whose horses are well broken, and whose reins are strong and kept well in the hands of the charioteer (the intellect) reaches the goal which is the state of Him, the Omnipresent. But the man whose horses (the senses) are not controlled, nor the reins (the mind) well-managed, goes to destruction. This Atman in all beings does not manifest Himself to the eyes or the senses, but those whose minds have become purified and refined realize Him. . . . He who realizes Him, frees himself from the jaws of death. (2:169–70)

Shaping One's Destiny

If it be true that we are working out our own destiny here within this short space of time, if it be true that everything must have a cause as we see it now, it must also be true that that which we are now is the effect of the whole of our past; therefore, no other person is necessary to shape the destiny of mankind but man himself. (2:242)

Knowledge can only be got in one way, the way of experience; there is no other way to know. If we have not experienced it in this life, we must have experienced it in other lives. (2:220)

Neither you, nor I, nor anyone present, has come out of zero, nor will go back to zero. We have been existing eternally, and will exist, and there is no power under the sun or above the sun which can undo your or my existence or send us back to zero. Now this idea of reincarnation is not only not a frightening idea, but is most essential for the moral well-being of the human race. (2:217)

No other theory except that of reincarnation accounts for the wide divergence that we find between man and man in their powers to acquire knowledge. (2:219)

Like fire in a piece of flint, knowledge exists in the mind; suggestion is the friction which brings it out. So with all our feelings and actions—our tears and our smiles, our joys and our griefs, our weeping and our laughter, our curses and our blessings, our praises and our blames—every one of these we may find, if we calmly study our own selves, to have been brought out from within ourselves by so many blows. The result is what we are. All these blows taken together are called karma—work, action. (1:28–29)

All search is vain, until we begin to perceive that knowledge is within ourselves, that no one can help us, that we must help ourselves. (1:258)

So what directs the soul when the body dies? The resultant, the sum total of all the works it has done, of the thoughts it has thought. If the resultant is such that it has to manufacture a new body for further experience, it will go to those parents who are ready to supply it with suitable material for that body. (2:223)

Basics

What is the watchword of all ethical codes? "Not I, but thou," and this "I" is the outcome of the Infinite that lies behind, trying to manifest Itself on the outside world. This little "I" is the result, and it will have to go back and join the Infinite, its own nature. Every time you say, "Not I, my brother, but thou," you are trying to go back, and every time you say, "I," and not "thou," you take the false step of trying to manifest the Infinite through the sense-world. That brings struggles and evils into the world, but after a time renunciation must come, eternal renunciation. The little "I" is dead and gone. (2:173)

Relative knowledge is good, because it leads to absolute knowledge; but neither the knowledge of the senses, nor of the mind, nor even of the Vedas is true, since they are all within the realm of relative knowledge. First get rid of the delusion "I am the body," then only can we want real knowledge. Man's knowledge is only a higher degree of brute knowledge. (7:33)

Each soul is potentially divine. The goal is to manifest this divinity within, by controlling nature, external and internal. Do this either by work, or worship, or psychic control, or philosophy— by one or more or all of these—and be free. This is the whole of religion. Doctrines, or dogmas, or rituals, or books, or temples, or forms, are but secondary details. (1:257)

In Each Dewdrop the Same Sun

The essence of Vedanta is that there is but one Being and that every soul is that Being in full, not a part of that Being. All the sun is reflected in each dewdrop. (8:6)

The ideal of Vedanta is that all wisdom and all purity are in the soul already, dimly expressed or better expressed—that is all the difference. The difference between man and man, and all things in the whole creation, is not in kind but only in degree. The background, the reality, of everyone is that same Eternal, Ever Blessed, Ever Pure, and Ever Perfect One. It is the Atman, the Soul, in the saint and the sinner, in the happy and the miserable, in the beautiful and the ugly, in men and in animals; it is the same throughout. It is the shining One. The difference is caused by the power of expression. In some It is expressed more, in others less, but this difference of expression has no effect upon the Atman. (2:168)

As manifested beings we appear to be separate, but our reality is one, and the less we think of ourselves as separate from that One, the better for us. The more we think of ourselves as separate from the Whole, the more miserable we become. From this monistic principle we get at the basis of ethics, and I venture to say that we cannot get any ethics from anywhere else. (2:334)

This is the basis of all ignorance that we, the immortal, the ever pure, the perfect Spirit, think that we are little minds, that we are little bodies; it is the mother of all selfishness. As soon as I think that I am a little body, I want to preserve it, to protect it, to keep it nice, at the expense of other bodies; then you and I become separate. As soon as this idea of separation comes, it opens the door to all mischief and leads to all misery. (2:83–84)

In reality, and at the back of all things, every being is equal. (6:128)

2

THE HUMAN CONDITION

The Forces of Good and Evil

If it is true that you cannot do good without doing evil, and whenever you try to create happiness there will always be misery, people will ask you, "What is the use of doing good?" The answer is, in the first place, that we must work for lessening misery, for that is the only way to make ourselves happy. Every one of us finds it out sooner or later in our lives. The bright ones find it out a little earlier, and the dull ones a little later. The dull ones pay very dearly for the discovery and the bright ones less dearly. In the second place, we must do our part, because that is the only way of getting out of this life of contradiction. Both the forces of good and evil will keep the universe alive for us, until we awake from our dreams and give up this building of mud pies. That lesson we shall have to learn, and it will take a long, long time to learn it. (2:98–99)

The evils that are in the world are caused by none else but ourselves. We have caused all this evil; and just as we constantly see misery resulting from evil actions, so can we also see that much of the existing misery in the world is the effect of the past wickedness of man. Man alone, therefore, according to this theory, is responsible. God is not to blame. (2:242)

The two conjoint facts of perception we can never get rid of are happiness and unhappiness—things which bring us pain also bring pleasure. Our world is made up of these two. We cannot get rid of them; with every pulsation of life they are present. The world is busy trying to reconcile these opposites, sages are busy trying to find the solution of this commingling of the opposites. (6:145)

Opposition to a righteous work initiated with moral courage will only awaken the moral power of the initiators the more. That which meets with no obstruction, no opposition, only takes men to the path of moral death. Struggle is the sign of life. (7:219)

Can any permanent happiness be given to the world? In the ocean we cannot raise a wave without causing a hollow somewhere else. The sum total of the good things in the world has been the same throughout in its relation to man's need and greed. It cannot be increased or decreased. (1:111)

A Nation's Well-Being

All growth, progress, well-being, or degradation is but relative. It refers to a certain standard, and each man to be understood has to be referred to that standard of his perfection. You see this more markedly in nations: what one nation thinks good might not be so regarded by another nation. (8:55)

The mythologists of all ancient races supply us with fables of heroes whose life was concentrated in a certain small portion of their bodies, and until that was touched they remained invulnerable. It seems as if each nation also has such a peculiar center of life, and so long as that remains untouched, no amount of misery and misfortune can destroy it. (4:324)

Each nation is a type, physically and mentally. Each is constantly receiving ideas from others only to work them *into* its type, that is, along the national line. The time has not come for the destruction of types. All education from any source is compatible with the ideals in every country; only they must be nationalized, i.e., fall in line with the rest of the type manifestation. (8:523–24)

There is a common platform, a common ground of understanding, a common humanity, which must be the basis of our work. We ought to find out that complete and perfect human nature which is working only in parts, here and there. It has not been given to one man to have everything in perfection. You have a part to play; I, in my humble way, another; here is one who plays a little part; there, another. The perfection is the combination of all these parts. Just as with individuals, so with races. Each race has a part to play; each race has one side of human nature to develop. And we have to take all these together; and, possibly in the distant future, some race will arise in which all these marvelous individual race perfections, attained by the different races, will come together and form a new race, the like of which the world has not yet dreamed. (8:56–57)

In each nation, man or woman represents an ideal consciously or unconsciously being worked out. The individual is the external expression of an ideal to be embodied. The collection of such individuals is the nation, which also represents a great ideal; toward that it is moving. And, therefore, it is rightly assumed that to understand a nation you must first understand its ideal, for each nation refuses to be judged by any other standard than its own. (8:55)

I am thoroughly convinced that no individual or nation can live by holding itself apart from the community of others, and whenever such an attempt has been made under false ideas of greatness, policy, or holiness—the result has always been disastrous to the secluding one. (4:365)

A nation may conquer the waves, control the elements, develop the utilitarian problems of life seemingly to the utmost limits, and yet not realize that in the individual, the highest type of civilization is found in him who has learned to conquer self. (4:200)

Truth does not pay homage to any society, ancient or modern. Society has to pay homage to Truth or die. Societies should be molded upon truth, and truth has not to adjust itself to society. (2:84)

You must bear in mind that religion has to do only with the soul and has no business to interfere in social matters; you must also bear in mind that this applies completely to the mischief which has already been done. It is as if a man after forcibly taking possession of another's property cries through the nose when that man tries to regain it—and preaches the doctrine of the sanctity of human right! (4:358–59)

Religion has no business to formulate social laws and insist on the difference between beings, because its aim and end is to obliterate all such fictions and monstrosities. (4:358)

In the Course of Human Events

This is the bane of human nature, the curse upon mankind, the root of all misery—this inequality. This is the source of all bondage, physical, mental, and spiritual. (4:329)

Meddle not with so-called social reform, for there cannot be any reform without spiritual reform first. (5:74)

The difficulty is not that one body of men are naturally more intelligent than another, but whether this body of men, because they have the advantage of intelligence, should take away even physical enjoyment from those who do not possess that advantage. The fight is to destroy that privilege. (1:435)

A redistribution of pain and pleasure is better than always the same persons having pains and pleasures. The sum total of good and evil in the world remains ever the same. The yoke will be lifted from shoulder to shoulder by new systems, that is all. (6:382)

Liberty does not certainly mean the absence of obstacles in the path of misappropriation of wealth, etc., by you and me, but it is our natural right to be allowed to use our own body, intelligence, or wealth according to our will, without doing any harm to others; and all the members of a society ought to have the same opportunity for obtaining wealth, education, or knowledge. (5:146)

We should never try to be guardians of mankind, or to stand on a pedestal as saints reforming sinners. Let us rather purify ourselves, and the result must be that in so doing we shall help others. (8:20)

When man has seen himself as one with the Infinite Being of the universe, when all separateness has ceased, when all men and women, all gods and angels, all animals and plants, and the whole universe have melted into that Oneness, then all fear disappears. (2:251–52)

Liberalism dies because it is dry, because it cannot rouse fanaticism in the human mind, because it cannot bring out hatred for everything except itself. That is why liberalism is bound to go down again and again. It can influence only small numbers of people. The reason is not hard to see. Liberalism tries to make us unselfish. But we do not want to be unselfish—we see no immediate gain in unselfishness; we gain more by being selfish. We accept liberalism as long as we are poor, have nothing. The moment we acquire money and power, we turn very conservative. The poor man is a democrat. When he becomes rich, he becomes an aristocrat. In religion, too, human nature acts in the same way. (8:123–24)

The word *toleration* has acquired an unpleasant association with the conceited man who, thinking himself in a high position, looks down on his fellow creatures with pity. This is a horrible state of mind. We are all traveling the same way, toward the same goal, but by different paths made by the necessities of the case to suit diverse minds. We must become many-sided, indeed we must become protean in character, so as not only to tolerate, but to do what is much more difficult, to sympathize, to enter into another's path, and feel *with him* in his aspirations and seeking after God. (6:137–38)

When a kettle of water is coming to the boil, if you watch the phenomenon, you find first one bubble rising, and then another and so on, until at last they all join, and a tremendous commotion takes place. This world is very similar. Each individual is like a bubble, and the nations resemble many bubbles. Gradually these nations are joining, and I am sure the day will come when separation will vanish and that Oneness to which we are all going will become manifest. A time must come when every man will be intensely practical in the scientific world and in the spiritual, and then that Oneness, the harmony of Oneness, will pervade the whole world. The whole of mankind will become jivanmuktas—free while living. We are all struggling toward that one end through our jealousies and hatreds, through our love and cooperation. A tremendous stream is flowing toward the ocean, carrying us all along with it; and though like straws and scraps of paper we may at times float aimlessly about, in the long run we are sure to join the Ocean of Life and Bliss. (2:187–88)

Make Yourself a Dynamo

We need to have three things; the heart to feel, the brain to conceive, the hand to work. First we must go out of the world and make ourselves fit instruments. Make yourself a dynamo. *Feel* first for the world. At a time when all men are ready to work, where is the man of *feeling*? . . . Test your love and humility. That man is not humble or loving who is jealous. Jealousy is a terrible, horrible sin; it enters a man so mysteriously. Ask yourself, does your mind react in hatred or jealousy? Good works are continually being undone by the tons of hatred and anger which are being poured out on the world. If you are pure, if you are strong, *you, one man*, are equal to the whole world. (6:144–45)

If in this hell of a world one can bring a little joy and peace even for a day into the heart of a single person, that much alone is true; this I have learnt after suffering all my life; all else is mere moonshine. (5:177)

The day will come when men will study history from a different light and find that competition is neither the cause nor the effect, simply a thing on the way, not necessary to evolution at all. (5:278)

The life of the married man is quite as great as that of the celibate who has devoted himself to religious work. The scavenger in the street is quite as great and glorious as the king on his throne. Take him off his throne, make him do the work of the scavenger, and see how he fares. Take up the scavenger and see how he will rule. It is useless to say that the man who lives out of the world is a greater man than he who lives in the world; it is much more difficult to live in the world and worship God than to give it up and live a free and easy life. (1:42)

It is the patient upbuilding of character, the intense struggle to *realize* the truth, which alone will tell in the future of humanity. (8:335)

Our principle should be love, and not compassion. The application of the word *compassion* even to jiva seems to me to be rash and vain. For us, it is not to pity but to serve. Ours is not the feeling of compassion but of love, and the feeling of Self in all. (5:133)

Perfect sincerity, holiness, gigantic intellect, and an all-conquering will. Let only a handful of men work with these, and the whole world will be revolutionized. (8:335)

3

THE INTENSE DESIRE
TO BE FREE

Freedom

He whom the sages have been seeking in all these places is in our own hearts; the voice that you heard was right, says the Vedanta, but the direction you gave to the voice was wrong. The ideal of freedom that you perceived was correct, but you projected it outside yourself, and that was your mistake. Bring it nearer and nearer, until you find that it was all the time within you, it was the Self of your own self. That freedom was your own nature, and this maya never bound you. (2:128)

The people of old knew that fire lived in the flint and in dry wood, but friction was necessary to call it out. So this fire of freedom and purity is the nature of every soul, and not a quality, because qualities can be acquired and therefore can be lost. The soul is one with Freedom, and the soul is one with Existence, and the soul is one with Knowledge. The Sat-Chit-Ananda—Existence-Knowledge-Bliss Absolute—is the nature, the birthright of the Soul, and all the manifestations that we see are Its expressions, dimly or brightly manifesting Itself. (2:193–94)

God is self-evident, impersonal, omniscient, the Knower and Master of nature, the Lord of all. He is behind all worship and it is being done according to Him, whether we know it or not. I go one step further. That at which all marvel, that which we call evil, is His worship too. This too is a part of freedom. Nay, I will be

LIVING AT THE SOURCE

terrible even and tell you that, when you are doing evil, the impulse behind is also that freedom. It may have been misguided and misled, but it was there; and there cannot be any life or any impulse unless that freedom be behind it. Freedom breathes in the throb of the universe. (1:337–38)

There is something in us which is free and permanent. . . . But it is not the body; neither is it the mind. The body is dying every minute. The mind is constantly changing. The body is a combination, and so is the mind, and as such can never reach to a state beyond all change. But beyond this momentary sheathing of gross matter, beyond even the finer covering of the mind is the Atman, the true Self of man, the permanent, the ever free. It is his freedom that is percolating through layers of thought and matter, and, in spite of the colorings of name and form, is ever asserting its unshackled existence. It is his deathlessness, his bliss, his peace, his divinity that shines out and makes itself felt in spite of the thickest layers of ignorance. He is the real man, the fearless one, the deathless one, the free. (4:256)

The soul cries ever, "Freedom, O Freedom!" With the conception of God as a perfectly free Being, man cannot rest eternally in this bondage. Higher he must go, and unless the struggle were for himself, he would think it too severe. Man says to himself, "I am a born slave, I am bound; nevertheless, there is a Being who is not bound by nature. He is free and Master of nature." The conception of God, therefore, is as essential and as fundamental a part of mind as is the idea of bondage. Both are the outcome of the idea of freedom. There cannot be life, even in the plant, without the idea of freedom. (1:335–36)

Freedom is the only condition of growth; take that off, the result is degeneration. (5:23)

Freedom and highest love must go together, then neither can become a bondage. (7:86)

We are all rushing toward freedom, we are all following that voice, whether we know it or not; as the children of the village were attracted by the music of the flute player, so we are all following the music of the voice without knowing it.

We are ethical when we follow that voice. Not only the human soul, but all creatures from the lowest to the highest have heard the voice and are rushing toward it; and in the struggle are either combining with each other or pushing each other out of the way. Thus come competition, joys, struggles, life, pleasure, and death, and the whole universe is nothing but the result of this mad struggle to reach the voice. This is the manifestation of nature.

What happens then? The scene begins to shift. As soon as you know the voice and understand what it is, the whole scene changes. The same world which was the ghastly battlefield of maya is now changed into something good and beautiful. We no longer curse nature, nor say that the world is horrible and that it is all vain; we need no longer weep and wail. As soon as we understand the voice, we see the reason why this struggle should be here, this fight, this competition, this difficulty, this cruelty, these little pleasures and joys; we see that they are in the nature of things, because without them there would be no going toward the voice, to attain which we are destined, whether we know it or not. All human life, all nature, therefore, is struggling to attain to freedom. (2:126–27)

The greatest goodness is the highest freedom. (6:100)

The One End to Be Attained

That action is moral which frees us from the bondage of matter and vice versa. This world appears infinite because everything is in a circle; it returns to whence it came. The circle meets, so there is no rest or peace here in any place. We must get out. Mukti is the one end to be attained. (7:102)

What is then worth having? Mukti, freedom. Even in the highest of heavens, says our scripture, you are a slave; what matters it if you are king for twenty thousand years? So long as you have a body, so long as you are a slave to happiness, so long as time works on you, space works on you, you are a slave. The idea, therefore, is to be free of external and internal nature. Nature must fall at your feet, and you must trample on it and be free and glorious by going beyond. No more is there life; therefore no more is there death. No more enjoyment; therefore no more misery. It is bliss unspeakable, indestructible, beyond everything. What we call happiness and good here are but particles of that eternal Bliss. And this eternal Bliss is our goal. (3:127–28)

In perfect concentration the soul becomes actually free from the bonds of the gross body and knows itself as it is. (4:226)

Desire, ignorance, and inequality—this is the trinity of bondage. (8:344)

The human soul has sojourned in lower and higher forms, migrating from one to another, according to the samskaras or impressions, but it is only in the highest form as man that it attains to freedom. (2:258)

Every action of man is worship, because the idea is to attain to freedom, and all action, directly or indirectly, tends to that. Only those actions that deter are to be avoided. The whole universe is worshiping, consciously or unconsciously; only it does not know that even while it is cursing, it is in another form worshiping the same God it is cursing, because those who are cursing are also struggling for freedom. (5:291)

The going from birth to death, this traveling, is what is called samsara in Sanskrit, the round of birth and death literally. All creation, passing through this round, will sooner or later become free. (2:259)

The Universal Cry

We want to know in order to make ourselves free. That is our life: one universal cry for freedom. (4:240)

When we have become free, we need not go mad and throw up society and rush off to die in the forest or the cave; we shall remain where we were, only we shall understand the whole thing. The same phenomena will remain, but with a new meaning. We do not know the world yet; it is only through freedom that we see what it is, and understand its nature. We shall see then that this so-called law or fate or destiny occupied only an infinitesimal part of our nature. It was only one side, but on the other side there was freedom all the time. We did not know this, and that is why we have been trying to save ourselves from evil by hiding our faces in the ground, like the hunted hare. Through delusion we have been trying to forget our nature, and yet we could not; it was always calling upon us, and all our search after God or gods, or external freedom, was a search after our real nature. We mistook the voice. (2:325)

All nature is crying through all the atoms for one thing—its perfect freedom. (4:241)

Pray all the time, read all the scriptures in the world, and worship all the gods there are . . . unless you realize the Soul there is no freedom. (4:245)

The universe itself can never be the limit of our satisfaction. That is why the miser gathers more and more money, that is why the robber robs, the sinner sins, that is why you are learning philosophy. All have one purpose. There is no other purpose in life, save to reach this freedom. Consciously or unconsciously, we are all striving for perfection. Every being must attain to it. (1:340)

We say that it is freedom that we are to seek, and that that freedom is God. It is the same happiness as in everything else; but when man seeks it in something which is finite, he gets only a spark of it. The thief when he steals gets the same happiness as the man who finds it in God; but the thief gets only a little spark with a mass of misery. The real happiness is God. Love is God, freedom is God; and everything that is bondage is not God. (5:288)

Strain Against the Bonds

The awakening of the soul to its bondage and its effort to stand up and assert itself—this is called life. Success in this struggle is called evolution. The eventual triumph, when all the slavery is blown away, is called salvation, nirvana, freedom. Everything in the universe is struggling for liberty. When I am bound by nature, by name and form, by time, space, and causality, I do not know what I truly am. But even in this bondage my real Self is not completely lost. I strain against the bonds; one by one they break, and I become conscious of my innate grandeur. Then comes complete liberation. I attain to the clearest and fullest consciousness of myself—I know that I am the infinite spirit, the master of nature, not its slave. Beyond all differentiation and combination, beyond space, time, and causation, I am that I am. (8:249)

The goal to be reached is freedom. I disagree with the idea that freedom is obedience to the laws of nature. I do not understand what that means. According to the history of human progress, it is disobedience to nature that has constituted that progress. (8:257)

This life is a tremendous assertion of freedom; excess of laws means death. (8:258)

To advance oneself toward freedom—physical, mental, and spiritual—and help others to do so, is the supreme prize of man. Those social rules which stand in the way of the unfoldment of this freedom are injurious, and steps should be taken to destroy them speedily. Those institutions should be encouraged by which men advance in the path of freedom. (5:147)

The Vedanta says that infinity is our true nature; it will never vanish, it will abide forever. But we are limiting ourselves by our karma, which like a chain round our necks has dragged us into this limitation. Break that chain and be free. Trample law under your feet. There is no law in human nature, there is no destiny, no fate. How can there be law in infinity? Freedom is its watchword. Freedom is its nature, its birthright. Be free, and then have any number of personalities you like. Then we will play like the actor who comes upon the stage and plays the part of a beggar. Contrast him with the actual beggar walking in the streets. The scene is, perhaps, the same in both cases, the words are, perhaps, the same, but yet what difference! The one enjoys his beggary while the other is suffering misery from it. And what makes this difference? The one is free and the other is bound. The actor knows his beggary is not true, but that he has assumed it for play, while the real beggar thinks that it is his too familiar state and that he has to bear it whether he wills it or not. This is the law. So long as we have no knowledge of our real nature, we are beggars, jostled about by every force in nature and made slaves of by everything in nature; we cry all over the world for help, but help never comes to us; we cry to imaginary beings, and yet it never comes. But still we hope help will come, and thus in weeping, wailing, and hoping, one life is passed, and the same play goes on and on. (2:323–24)

The Struggle Toward Freedom

There is to be found in every religion the manifestation of this struggle toward freedom. It is the groundwork of all morality, of unselfishness, which means getting rid of the idea that men are the same as their little body. (1:109)

If a piece of burning charcoal be placed on a man's head, see how he struggles to throw it off. Similar will be the struggles for freedom of a man who really understands that he is a slave of nature. (1:411)

Man must have education. They speak of democracy, of the equality of all men, these days. But how will a man know he is equal with all? He must have a strong brain, a clear mind free of nonsensical ideas; he must pierce through the mass of superstitions encrusting his mind to the pure truth that is in his inmost Self. Then he will know that all perfections, all powers are already within himself, that these have not to be given him by others. When he realizes this, he becomes free that moment, he achieves equality. He also realizes that everyone else is equally as perfect as he, and he does not have to exercise any power, physical, mental, or moral, over his brother men. He abandons the idea that there was ever any man who was lower than himself. Then he can talk of equality; not until then. (8:94)

If you think that you are bound, you remain bound; you make your own bondage. If you know that you are free, you are free this moment. This is knowledge, knowledge of freedom. Freedom is the goal of all nature. (2:462)

So long as there is desire or want, it is a sure sign that there is imperfection. A perfect, free being cannot have any desire. (2:261)

The monkeys of Varanasi [Benares] are huge brutes and are sometimes surly. They now took it into their heads not to allow me to pass through their street, so they howled and shrieked and clutched at my feet as I passed. As they pressed closer, I began to run, but the faster I ran, the faster came the monkeys and they began to bite at me. It seemed impossible to escape, but just then I met a stranger who called out to me, "Face the brutes." I turned and faced the monkeys, and they fell back and finally fled. That is a lesson for all life—face the terrible, face it boldly. Like the monkeys, the hardships of life fall back when we cease to flee before them. If we are ever to gain freedom, it must be by conquering nature, never by running away. Cowards never win victories. We have to fight fear and troubles and ignorance if we expect them to flee before us. (1:338–39)

The moment I have realized God sitting in the temple of every human body, the moment I stand in reverence before every human being and see God in him—that moment I am free from bondage, everything that binds vanishes, and I am free. (2:321)

We are ever free if we would only believe it, only have faith enough. You are the soul, free and eternal, ever free, ever blessed. Have faith enough and you will be free in a minute. (6:93)

Our sole concern is to know the highest truth. Our goal is the loftiest. We have said big words to ourselves—absolute realization and all that. Let us measure up to the words. Let us worship the spirit in spirit, standing on spirit. Let the foundation be spirit, the middle spirit, the culmination spirit. There will be no world anywhere. Let it go and whirl into space—who cares? Stand thou in the spirit! That is the goal. We know we cannot reach it yet. Never mind. Do not despair, and do not drag the ideal down. The important thing is: how much less you think of the body, of yourself as matter—as dead, dull, insentient matter; how much more you think of yourself as shining immortal being. The more you think of yourself as shining immortal spirit, the more eager you will be to be absolutely free of matter, body, and senses. This is the intense desire to be free. (8:120)

4

NO ONE IS AN ISLAND

The Luminous Idea

The one great idea that to me seems to be clear, and comes out through masses of superstition in every country and in every religion, is the one luminous idea that man is divine, that divinity is our nature. (2:193)

When you look at that unchanging Existence from the outside, you call it God; and when you look at it from the inside, you call it yourself. It is but one. There is no God separate from you, no God higher than you, the real "you." All the gods are little beings to you, all the ideas of God and Father in heaven are but your own reflections. God Himself is your image. (3:24)

One idea seems to be common in all the Indian systems, and I think, in every system in the world, whether they know it or not, and that is what I should call the divinity of man. There is no one system in the world, no real religion, which does not hold the idea that the human soul, whatever it be, or whatever its relation to God, is essentially pure and perfect, whether expressed in the language of mythology, allegory, or philosophy. Its real nature is blessedness and power, not weakness and misery. Somehow or other this misery has come. (2:193)

We attend lectures and read books, argue and reason about God and soul, religion and salvation. These are not spirituality, because spirituality does not exist in books or in theories or in philosophies.

It is not in learning or reasoning, but in actual inner growth. Even parrots can learn things by heart and repeat them. If you become learned, what of it? Asses can carry whole libraries. So when real light will come, there will be no more of this learning from books— no book-learning. The man who cannot write even his own name can be perfectly religious, and the man with all the libraries of the world in his head may fail to be. Learning is not a condition of spiritual growth; scholarship is not a condition. The touch of the guru, the transmittal of spiritual energy, will quicken your heart. Then will begin the growth. That is the real baptism by fire. (8:114)

The yogis say that man can go beyond his direct sense-perception, and beyond his reason also. Man has in him the faculty, the power, of transcending his intellect even, a power which is in every being, every creature. By the practice of yoga that power is aroused, and then man transcends the ordinary limits of reason, and directly perceives things which are beyond all reason. (1:232-33)

The first sign that you are becoming religious is that you are becoming cheerful. When a man is gloomy, that may be dyspepsia, but it is not religion. (1:264)

My noble Prince, this life is short, the vanities of the world are transient, but they alone live who live for others, the rest are more dead than alive. (4:363)

The work of ethics has been, and will be in the future, not the destruction of variation and the establishment of sameness in the external world—which is impossible for it would bring death and annihilation—but to recognize the unity in spite of all these variations, to recognize the God within, in spite of everything that frightens us, to recognize that infinite strength as the property of everyone in spite of all apparent weakness, and to recognize the eternal, infinite, essential purity of the soul in spite of everything to the contrary that appears on the surface. (1:436)

Keeping Your Balance

No sooner a prophet feels miserable for the state of man than he sours his face, beats his breast, and calls upon everyone to drink tartaric acid, munch charcoal, sit upon a dungheap covered with ashes, and speak only in groans and tears! (7:521)

We must be bright and cheerful, long faces do not make religion. Religion should be the most joyful thing in the world, because it is the best. . . . The essential thing in religion is making the heart pure; the Kingdom of Heaven is within us, but only the pure in heart can see the King. While we think of the world, it is only the world for us; but let us come to it with the feeling that the world is God, and we shall have God. (8:7–8)

I know full well how good it is for one's worldly prospects to be *sweet*. I do everything to be *sweet*, but when it comes to a horrible compromise with the truth within, then I stop. (5:70)

Combine seriousness with childlike naiveté. Live in harmony with all. (6:329)

Every wave of passion restrained is a balance in your favor. It is therefore good *policy* not to return anger for anger, as with all true morality. (6:136)

The chaste brain has tremendous energy and gigantic willpower. Without chastity there can be no spiritual strength. (1:263)

We should cultivate the optimistic temperament, and endeavor to see the good that dwells in everything. If we sit down and lament over the imperfection of our bodies and minds, we profit nothing; it is the heroic endeavor to subdue adverse circumstances that carries our spirit upward. (4:190)

This mind, so deluded, so weak, so easily led, even this mind can be strong and may catch a glimpse of that knowledge, that Oneness, which saves us from dying again and again. As rain falling upon a mountain flows in various streams down the sides of the mountain, so all the energies which you see here are from that one Unit. It has become manifold falling upon maya. Do not run after the manifold; go toward the One. (2:182)

In judging others we always judge them by our own ideals. That is not as it should be. Everyone must be judged according to his own ideal, and not by that of anyone else. (2:105–6)

Intellectual gymnastics are necessary at first. We must not go blindly into anything. The yogi has passed the argumentative state, and has come to a conclusion, which is, like the rocks, immovable. (1:236)

Books are infinite in number, and time is short; therefore the secret of knowledge is to take what is essential. Take that and try to live up to it. (1:236)

Excessive merriment will always be followed by sorrow. Tears and laughter are near kin. People so often run from one extreme to the other. Let the mind be cheerful, but calm. Never let it run into excesses, because every excess will be followed by a reaction. (4:11)

Negating the Negatives

In criticizing another, we always foolishly take one especially brilliant point as the whole of our life and compare that with the dark ones in the life of another. Thus we make mistakes in judging individuals. (5:267)

A yogi must not think of injuring anyone by thought, word, or deed. Mercy shall not be for men alone, but shall go beyond, and embrace the whole world. (1:137)

Never talk about the faults of others, no matter how bad they may be. Nothing is ever gained by that. You never help one by talking about his fault; you do him an injury, and injure yourself as well. (6:127)

Bless men when they revile you. Think how much good they are doing by helping to stamp out the false ego. Hold fast to the real Self, think only pure thoughts, and you will accomplish more than a regiment of mere preachers. Out of purity and silence comes the word of power. (8:31–32)

Blame neither man, nor God, nor anyone in the world. When you find yourselves suffering, blame yourselves, and try to do better. (2:225)

You must not criticize others; you must criticize *yourself*. If you see a drunkard, do not criticize him; remember he is you in another shape. He who has not darkness sees no darkness in others. What you have inside you is that which you see in others. This is the surest way of reform. If the would-be reformers who criticize and see evil would themselves stop creating evil, the world would be better. Beat this idea into yourself. (6:129)

Whatever others think or do, lower not your standard of purity, morality, and love of God. (8:382)

Come to God any way you can; only come. But in coming do not push anyone down. (7:97)

The world has its code of judgment which, alas, is very different from that of truth's. (8:414)

Though they all believe in immortality, they do not know that immortality is not gained by dying and going to heaven, but by giving up this piggish individuality, by not tying ourselves down to one little body. Immortality is knowing ourselves as one with all, living in all bodies, perceiving through all minds. We are bound to feel in other bodies than this one. We are bound to feel in other bodies. What is sympathy? Is there any limit to this sympathy, this feeling in our bodies? It is quite possible that the time will come when I shall feel through the whole universe. (8:130)

Securing One's Own Good

I can secure my own good only by doing you good. There is no other way, none whatsoever. . . . You are God, I am God, and man is God. It is this God manifested through humanity who is doing everything in this world. Is there a different God sitting high up somewhere? To work, therefore! (6:317)

Doing good to others is the one great, universal religion. (6:403)

It is only by doing good to others that one attains to one's own good. (6:266)

Our duty to others means helping others; doing good to the world. Why should we do good to the world? Apparently to help the world, but really to help ourselves. (1:75)

Devotion to the mother is the root of all welfare. (8:530)

Do not stand on a high pedestal and take five cents in your hand and say, "Here, my poor man," but be grateful that the poor man is there, so that by making a gift to him you are able to help yourself. It is not the receiver that is blessed, but it is the giver. (1:76)

Manifest the divinity within you, and everything will be harmoniously arranged around it. (4:351)

By being nervous and fearful we injure others. By being so fearful to hurt we hurt more. By trying so much to avoid evil we fall into its jaws. (6:429)

If you are a strong man, very good! But do not curse others who are not strong enough for you. . . . Everyone says, "Woe unto you people!" Who says, "Woe unto me that I cannot help you"? The people are doing all right to the best of their ability and means and knowledge. Woe unto me that I cannot lift them to where I am! (1:439)

Love All Alike

To love anyone personally is bondage. Love all alike, then all desires fall off. (7:66)

What we are, we see outside, for the world is our mirror. This little body is a little mirror we have created, but the whole universe is our body. We must think this all the time; then we shall know that we cannot die or hurt another, because he is our own. We are birthless and deathless and we ought only to love. (8:48–49)

With the love of God will come, as a sure effect, the love of everyone in the universe. The nearer we approach God, the more do we begin to see that all things are in Him. When the soul succeeds in appropriating the bliss of this supreme love, it also begins to see Him in everything. Our heart will thus become an eternal fountain of love. (3:82)

Love for love's sake cannot be expressed to those who have not felt it. (6:143)

Many feel, but only a few can express. It is the power of expressing one's love and appreciation and sympathy for others, that enables one person to succeed better in spreading the idea than others. (8:428–29)

The world cares little for principles. They care for persons. They will hear with patience the words of a man they like, however nonsensical, and will not listen to anyone they do not like. Think of this and modify your conduct accordingly. Everything will come all right. Be the servant if you will rule. That is the real secret. Your love will tell even if your words be harsh. Instinctively men feel the love clothed in whatever language. (7:482–83)

We hear so much tall talk in this world, of liberal ideas and sympathy with differences of opinion. That is very good, but as a fact, we find that one sympathizes with another only so long as the other believes in everything one has to say, but as soon as he dares to differ, that sympathy is gone, that love vanishes. (3:208)

Know partiality to be the chief cause of all evil. That is to say, if you show toward anyone more love than toward somebody else, rest assured, you will be sowing the seeds of future troubles. . . . Moreover, bear with everyone's shortcomings. Forgive offenses by the million. And if you love all unselfishly, all will by degrees come to love one another. (6:322–23)

We believe that it is the duty of every *soul* to treat, think of, and behave to other *souls* as such, i.e., as *Gods*, and not hate or despise, or vilify, or try to injure them by any manner of means. (4:357)

The Only True Teacher

The only true teacher is he who can immediately come down to the level of the student, and transfer his soul to the student's soul and see through the student's eyes and hear through his ears and understand through his mind. (4:183)

As soon as the soul earnestly desires to have religion, the transmitter of the religious force *must* and does appear to help that soul. (3:46)

How is harmonious development of character to be best effected? By association with persons whose character has been so developed. (5:315)

Get the mercy of God and of His greatest children; these are the two chief ways to God. The company of these children of light is very hard to get; five minutes in their company will change a whole life; and if you really want it enough, one will come to you. The presence of those who love God makes a place holy, "such is the glory of the children of the Lord." They are He; and when they speak, their words are scriptures. The place where they have been becomes filled with their vibrations, and those going there feel them and have a tendency to become holy also. (7:10)

The disciple must have faith in the guru (teacher). In the West the teacher simply gives intellectual knowledge; that is all. The relationship with the teacher is the greatest in life. My dearest and nearest relative in life is my guru; next, my mother; then my father. My first reverence is to the guru. If my father says, "Do this," and my guru says, "Do not do this," I do not do it. The guru frees my soul. The father and mother give me this body; but the guru gives me rebirth in the soul. (8:112)

When through the guru's instructions and your own conviction you will see, not this world of name and form, but the essence which lies as its substratum, then only you will realize your identity with the whole universe from the Creator down to a clump of grass, then only you will get the state in which "the knots of the heart are cut asunder and all doubts are dispelled." (7:164)

The guru must teach me and lead me into light, make me a link in that chain of which he himself is a link. The man in the street cannot claim to be a guru. The guru must be a man who has known, has actually realized the divine truth, has perceived himself as the spirit. A mere talker cannot be the guru. (8:115)

The *sine qua non* of acquiring spiritual truth for one's self or for imparting it to others is the purity of heart and soul. (3:50)

A leader must be impersonal. I am sure you understand this. I do not mean that one should be a brute, making use of the devotion of others for his own ends, and laughing in his sleeve meanwhile. What I mean is what I am, intensely personal in my love, but having the power to pluck out my own heart with my own hand, if it becomes necessary, "for the good of many, for the welfare of many," as Buddha said. Madness of love, and yet in it no bondage. (8:429)

You are the greatest book that ever was or ever will be, the infinite depository of all that is. Until the inner teacher opens, all outside teaching is in vain. It must lead to the opening of the book of the heart to have any value. (7:71)

How are we to know a teacher then? In the first place, the sun requires no torch to make it visible. We do not light a candle to see the sun. When the sun rises, we instinctively become aware of its rising; and when a teacher of men comes to help us, the soul will instinctively know that it has found the truth. Truth stands on its own evidences; it does not require any other testimony to attest it; it is self-effulgent. It penetrates into the inmost recesses of our nature, and the whole universe stands up and says, "This is Truth." (4:23–24)

5

SO MANY PEOPLE,
SO MANY PATHS

To See for Yourself

In order to prove religion—that is, the existence of God, immortality, etc.—we have to go beyond the knowledge of the senses. All great prophets and seers claim to have "seen God," that is to say, they have had direct experience. There is no knowledge without experience, and man has to see God in his own soul. When man has come face to face with the one great fact in the universe, then alone will doubts vanish and crooked things become straight. This is "seeing God." Our business is to verify, now to swallow. Religion, like other sciences, requires you to gather facts, to see for yourself, and this is possible when you go beyond the knowledge which lies in the region of the five senses. Religious truths need verification by everyone. To see God is the one goal. (6:132–33)

Religion does not consist in doctrines or dogmas. It is not what you read, nor what dogmas you believe that is of importance, but what you realize. "Blessed are the pure in heart, for they shall see God," yea, in this life. And that is salvation. There are those who teach that this can be gained by the mumbling of words. But no great Master ever taught that external forms were necessary for salvation. The power of attaining it is within ourselves. We live and move in God. Creeds and sects have their parts to play, but they are for children, they last but temporarily. Books never make religions, but religions make books. We must not forget that. No book ever created God, but God inspired all the great books. And no book ever created a soul. We must never forget that. The end of all religions is the realizing of God in the soul. That is the one universal religion. If there is one universal truth in all religions, I place it here—in realizing God. Ideals and methods may differ, but that is the central point. (1:324–25)

All pleasures of the senses or even of the mind are evanescent, but within ourselves is the one true unrelated pleasure, dependent on nothing outside. "The pleasure of the Self is what the world calls religion." (8:29)

Each religion brings out its own doctrines and insists upon them as being the only true ones. And not only does it do that, but it thinks that he who does not believe in them must go to some horrible place. Some will even draw the sword to compel others to believe as they do. This is not through wickedness, but through a particular disease of the human brain called fanaticism. They are very sincere, these fanatics, the most sincere of human beings; but they are quite as irresponsible as other lunatics in the world. This disease of fanaticism is one of the most dangerous of all diseases. All the wickedness of human nature is roused by it. Anger is stirred up, nerves are strung high, and human beings become like tigers. (2:377–78)

Are all the religions of the world really contradictory? I do not mean the external forms in which great thoughts are clad. I do not mean the different buildings, languages, rituals, books, etc., employed in various religions, but I mean the internal soul of every religion. I believe that they are not contradictory; they are supplementary. Each religion, as it were, takes up one part of the great universal truth, and spends its whole force in embodying and typifying that part of the great truth. (2:365)

Now, as regards those of you that think that you understand truth and divinity and God in only one Prophet in the world, and not in any other, naturally, the conclusion which I draw is that you do not understand divinity in anybody; you have simply swallowed words and identified yourself with one sect, just as you would in party politics, as a matter of opinion; but that is no religion at all. There are some fools in this world who use brackish water although there is excellent sweet water nearby, because, they say, the brack-ish-water well was dug by their father. Now, in my little experience I have collected this knowledge—that for all the devilry that religion is blamed with, religion is not at all in fault; no religion ever persecuted men, no religion ever burnt witches, no religion ever did any of these things. What then incited people to do these things? Politics, but never religion; and if such politics takes the name of religion whose fault is that?

So, when each man stands and says, "My prophet is the only true prophet," he is not correct—he knows not the alpha of religion. Religion is neither talk, nor theory, nor intellectual con-sent. It is realization in the heart of our hearts; it is touching God; it is feeling, realizing that I am a spirit in relation with the Universal Spirit and all Its great manifestations. (4:125–26)

Experience is the only source of knowledge. In the world, religion is the only science where there is no surety, because it is not taught as a science of experience. This should not be. There is always, however, a small group of men who teach religion from experience. They are called mystics, and these mystics in every religion speak the same tongue and teach the same truth. This is the real science of religion. As mathematics in every part of the world does not differ, so the mystics do not differ. They are all similarly consti-tuted and similarly situated. Their experience is the same; and this becomes law. (6:81)

If there ever is going to be an ideal religion, it must be broad and large enough to supply food for all these minds. It must supply the strength of philosophy to the philosopher, the devotee's heart to the worshiper; to the ritualist, it will give all that the most marvel-ous symbolism can convey; to the poet, it will give as much of heart as he can take in, and other things besides. To make such a broad religion, we shall have to go back to the time when religions began and take them all in.

Our watchword, then, will be acceptance, and not exclusion. Not only toleration, for so-called toleration is often blasphemy, and I do not believe in it. I believe in acceptance. (2:373–74)

The Man, the Buffalo, and the Fish

If the buffaloes desire to worship God, they, in keeping with their own nature, will see Him as a huge buffalo; if a fish wishes to worship God, its concept of Him would inevitably be a big fish; and man must think of Him as man. Suppose man, the buffalo, and the fish represent so many different vessels; that these vessels all go to the sea of God to be filled, each according to its shape and capacity. In man the water takes the shape of man; in the buffalo the shape of the buffalo; and in the fish the shape of the fish; but in each of these vessels is the same water of the sea of God. (8:256)

All who have actually attained any real religious nature never wrangle over the form in which the different religions are expressed. They know that the life of all religions is the same, and, consequently, they have no quarrel with anybody because he does not speak the same tongue. (6:47)

The ultimate goal of all mankind, the aim and end of all religions, is but one—reunion with God, or, what amounts to the same, with the divinity which is every man's true nature. But while the aim is one, the method of attaining may vary with the different temperaments of men. (5:292)

We cannot imagine anything which is not God. He is all that we can imagine with our five senses, and more. He is like a chameleon; each man, each nation, sees one face of Him and at different times, in different forms. Let each man see and take of God whatever is suitable to him. Compare each animal absorbing from nature whatever food is suitable to it. (6:120)

39

The Infinite Being we see from different standpoints, from different planes of mind. The lowest man sees Him as an ancestor; as his vision gets higher, as the governor of a planet; still higher as the governor of the universe, and the highest man sees Him as himself. It was the same God, and the different realizations were only degrees and differences of vision. (8:189)

The varieties of religious belief are an advantage, since all faiths are good, so far as they encourage man to lead a religious life. The more sects there are, the more opportunities there are for making successful appeals to the divine instinct in all men. (5:292)

When a number of people from various angles and distances have a look at the sea, each man sees a portion of it according to his horizon. Though each man may say that what he sees is the real sea, all of them speak the truth, for all of them see portions of the same wide expanse. So the religious scriptures, though they seem to contain varying and conflicting statements, speak the truth, for they are all descriptions of that one infinite Reality. (6:103–4)

To learn this central secret that the truth may be one and yet many at the same time, that we may have different visions of the same truth from different standpoints, is exactly what must be done. Then, instead of antagonism to anyone, we shall have infinite sympathy with all. Knowing that as long as there are different natures born in this world, the same religious truth will require different adaptations, we shall understand that we are bound to have forbearance with each other. (4:181)

It has been recognized in the most ancient times that there are various forms of worshiping God. It is also recognized that different natures require different methods. Your method of coming to God may not be my method, possibly it might hurt me. Such an idea as that there is but one way for everybody is injurious, meaningless, and entirely to be avoided. Woe unto the world when everyone is of the same religious opinion and takes to the same path. Then all religions and all thought will be destroyed. Variety is the very soul of life. When it dies out entirely, creation will die. When this variation in thought is kept up, we must exist; and we need not quarrel because of that variety. Your way is very good for you, but not for me. My way is good for me but not for you. (3:131)

But so long as mankind thinks, there will be sects. Variation is the sign of life, and it must be there. I pray that they may multiply so that at last there will be as many sects as human beings, and each one will have his own method, his individual method of thought in religion. (2:364)

I shall go to the mosque of the Muslim; I shall enter the Christian's church and kneel before the crucifix; I shall enter the Buddhistic temple, where I shall take refuge in Buddha and in his Law. I shall go into the forest and sit down in meditation with the Hindu, who is trying to see the Light which enlightens the heart of everyone. Not only shall I do all these, but I shall keep my heart open for all that may come in the future. Is God's book finished? Or is it still a continuous revelation going on? (2:374)

I may not find it when I try to grasp it, to sense it, and to actualize it, yet I know for certain that it is there. If I am sure of anything, it is of this humanity which is common to us all. It is through this generalized entity that I see you as a man or a woman. So it is with this universal religion, which runs through all the various religions of the world in the form of God; it must and does exist through eternity. "I am the thread that runs through all these pearls," and each pearl is a religion or even a sect thereof. Such are the different pearls, and the Lord is the thread that runs through all of them; only the majority of mankind are entirely unconscious of it. (2:381)

The language of the soul is one, the languages of nations are many; their customs and methods of life are widely different.

Religion is of the soul and finds expression through various nations, languages, and customs. Hence it follows that the difference between the religions of the world is one of expression and not of substance; and their points of similarity and unity are of the soul, are intrinsic, as the language of the soul is one, in whatever peoples and under whatever circumstances it manifests itself. The same sweet harmony is vibrant there also, as it is on many and diverse instruments. (6:46)

Realizing the Spirit

Worship of the Impersonal God is through truth. And what is truth? That I am He. When I say that I am not Thou, it is untrue. When I say I am separate from you, it is a lie, a terrible lie. I am one with this universe, born one. It is self-evident to my senses that I am one with the universe. I am one with the air that surrounds me, one with heat, one with light, eternally one with the whole Universal Being, who is called this universe, who is mistaken for the universe, for it is He and nothing else, the eternal subject in the heart who says, "I am," in every heart—the deathless one, the sleepless one, ever awake, the immortal, whose glory never dies, whose powers never fail. I am one with That. (1:380–81)

This is the message of Shri Ramakrishna to the modern world: "Do not care for doctrines, do not care for dogmas, or sects, or churches, or temples; they count for little compared with the essence of existence in each man, which is spirituality; and the more this is developed in a man, the more powerful is he for good. Earn that first, acquire that, and criticize no one, for all doctrines and creeds have some good in them. Show by your lives that religion does not mean words, or names, or sects, but that it means spiritual realization. Only those can understand who have felt. Only those who have attained to spirituality can communicate it to others, can be great teachers of mankind. They alone are the powers of light." (4:187)

With the thirst, the longing for God, comes real devotion, real bhakti. Who has the longing? That is the question. Religion is not in doctrines, in dogmas, nor in intellectual argumentation; it is being and becoming, it is realization. We hear so many talking about God and the soul, and all the mysteries of the universe, but if you take them one by one, and ask them, "Have you realized God? Have you seen your Soul?"—how many can say they have? And yet they are all fighting with one another! (2:43)

Although a man has not studied a single system of philosophy, although he does not believe in any God, and never has believed, although he has not prayed even once in his whole life, if the simple power of good actions has brought him to that state where he is ready to give up his life and all else for others, he has arrived at the same point to which the religious man will come through his prayers and the philosopher through his knowledge; and so you may find that the philosopher, the worker, and the devotee, all meet at one point, that one point being self-abnegation. (1:86)

All the means we take to reach God are true; it is only like trying to find the pole-star by locating it through the stars that are around it. (7:57)

It is a degradation to worship God through fear of punishment; such worship is, if worship at all, the crudest form of the worship of love. So long as there is any fear in the heart, how can there be love also? Love conquers naturally all fear. (3:88)

Realization of the truth is the essential thing. Whether you bathe in the Ganga for a thousand years or live on vegetable food for a like period, unless it helps toward the manifestation of the Self, know that it is all of no use. If, on the other hand, anyone can realize the Atman without the observance of outward forms, then that very nonobservance of forms is the best means. (7:210–11)

The Lord is the great magnet, and we are all like iron filings; we are being constantly attracted by Him, and all of us are struggling to reach Him. All this struggling of ours in this world is surely not intended for selfish ends. Fools do not know what they are doing; the work of their life is, after all, to approach the great magnet. All the tremendous struggling and fighting in life is intended to make us go to Him ultimately and be one with Him. (3:75)

Through high philosophy or low, through the most exalted mythology or the grossest, through the most refined ritualism or arrant fetishism, every sect, every soul, every nation, every religion, consciously or unconsciously, is struggling upward, toward God; every vision of truth that man has, is a vision of Him and of none else. (2:383)

Like the Tide Rushing

No bhakta cares for anything except love, except to love and to be loved. His unworldly love is like the tide rushing up the river; this lover goes up the river against the current. The world calls him mad. I know one whom the world used to call mad, and this was his answer: "My friends, the whole world is a lunatic asylum. Some are mad after worldly love, some after name, some after fame, some after money, some after salvation and going to heaven. In this big lunatic asylum I am also mad, I am mad after God. If you are mad after money, I am mad after God. You are mad; so am I. I think my madness is after all the best." (3:99–100)

The perfected bhakta no more goes to see God in temples and churches; he knows no place where he will not find Him. He finds Him in the temple as well as out of the temple, he finds Him in the saint's saintliness as well as in the wicked man's wickedness. (3:92)

When this supreme love once comes into the heart of man, his mind will continuously think of God and remember nothing else. He will give no room in himself to thoughts other than those of God, and his soul will be unconquerably pure and will alone break all the bonds of mind and matter and become serenely free. He alone can worship the Lord in his own heart; to him forms, symbols, books, and doctrines are all unnecessary and are incapable of proving serviceable in any way. It is not easy to love the Lord thus. (3:86)

But those to whom the eternal interests of the soul are of much higher value than the fleeting interests of this mundane life, to whom the gratification of the senses is but like the thoughtless play of the baby, to them God and the love of God form the highest and the only utility of human existence. Thank God there are some such still living in this world of too much worldliness. (3:43)

That religious ferment, which at present is every day gaining a greater hold over thinking men, has this characteristic—that all the little thought-whirlpools into which it has broken itself declare one single aim, a vision and a search after the Unity of Being. (8:347)

As our human relations can be made divine, so our relationship with God may take any of these forms and we can look upon Him as our father, or mother, or friend, or beloved. Calling God Mother is a higher ideal than calling Him Father; and to call Him Friend is still higher; but the highest is to regard Him as the Beloved. The highest point of all is to see no difference between lover and beloved. (2:326)

The goal of all nature is freedom, and freedom is to be attained only by perfect unselfishness; every thought, word, or deed that is unselfish takes us toward the goal, and, as such, is called moral. That definition, you will find, holds good in every religion and every system of ethics. In some systems of thought morality is derived from a Superior Being—God. If you ask why a man ought to do this and not that, their answer is: "Because such is the command of God." But whatever be the source from which it is derived, their code of ethics also has the same central idea—not to think of self but to give up self. (1:110)

There are moments when every man feels that he is one with the universe, and he rushes forth to express it, whether he knows it or not. This expression of oneness is what we call love and sympathy, and it is the basis of all our ethics and morality. This is summed up in the Vedanta philosophy by the celebrated aphorism *Tat tvam asi*, "Thou art That." (1:389)

A still higher stage of love is reached when life itself is maintained for the sake of the one ideal of Love, when life itself is considered beautiful and worth living only on account of that Love. Without it, such a life would not remain even for a moment. Life is sweet, because it thinks of the Beloved. (3:80)

6

EFFORTS IN
SELF-DISCOVERY

Nurturing Faith in Oneself

Throughout the history of mankind, if any motive power has been more potent than another in the lives of all great men and women, it is that of faith in themselves. Born with the consciousness that they were to be great, they became great. Let a man go down as low as possible; there must come a time when out of sheer desperation he will take an upward curve and will learn to have faith in himself. But it is better for us that we should know it from the very first. Why should we have all these bitter experiences in order to gain faith in ourselves? We can see that all the difference between man and man is owing to the existence or nonexistence of faith in himself. Faith in ourselves will do everything. . . . The old religions said that he was an atheist who did not believe in God. The new religion says that he is the atheist who does not believe in himself. (2:301)

The remedy for weakness is not brooding over weakness, but thinking of strength. Teach men of the strength that is already within them. Instead of telling them they are sinners, the Vedanta takes the opposite position and says, "You are pure and perfect, and what you call sin does not belong to you." Sins are very low degrees of Self-manifestation; manifest your Self in a high degree. That is the one thing to remember; all of us can do that. Never say, "No," never say, "I cannot," for you are infinite. Even time and

47

space are as nothing compared with your nature. You can do anything and everything, you are almighty. (2:300)

What makes you weak? What makes you fear? You are the One Being in the universe. What frightens you? Stand up then and be free. Know that every thought and word that weakens you in this world is the only evil that exists. Whatever makes men weak and makes them fear is the only evil that should be shunned. (2:236)

Virtue is that which tends to our improvement, and vice to our degeneration. Man is made up of three qualities—brutal, human, and godly. That which tends to increase the divinity in you is virtue, and that which tends to increase brutality in you is vice. You must kill the brutal nature and become human, that is, loving and charitable. You must transcend that too and become pure bliss—Sat-Chit-Ananda, fire without burning, wonderfully loving, but without the weakness of human love, without the feeling of misery. (6:112)

Religion gives you nothing new; it only takes off obstacles and lets you see your Self. Sickness is the first great obstacle; a healthy body is the best instrument. Melancholy is an almost insuperable barrier. If you have once known Brahman, never after can you be melancholy. Doubt, want of perseverance, mistaken ideas are other obstacles. (7:62)

Perfect morality is the all in all of complete control over mind. The man who is perfectly moral has nothing more to do; he is free. The man who is perfectly moral cannot possibly hurt anything or anybody. Non-injuring has to be attained by him who would be free. No one is more powerful than he who has attained perfect non-injuring. No one could fight, no one could quarrel, in his presence. Yes, his very presence, and nothing else, means peace, means love wherever he may be. Nobody could be angry or fight in his presence. Even the animals, ferocious animals, would be peaceful before him. (6:126)

No man should be judged by his defects. The great virtues a man has are his especially, his errors are the common weaknesses of humanity and should never be counted in estimating his character. (7:78)

Awakenings

Every soul is destined to be perfect, and every being, in the end, will attain the state of perfection. Whatever we are now is the result of our acts and thoughts in the past; and whatever we shall be in the future will be the result of what we think and do now. But this, the shaping of our destinies, does not preclude our receiving help from outside; nay, in the vast majority of cases such help is absolutely necessary. When it comes, the higher powers and possibilities of the soul are quickened, spiritual life is awakened, growth is animated, and man becomes holy and perfect in the end. (3:45)

Until the superconscious opens for you, religion is mere talk, it is nothing but preparation. You are talking secondhand, thirdhand. (3:253–54)

No book, no person, no Personal God. All these must go. Again, the senses must go. We cannot be bound to the senses. At present we are tied down—like persons dying of cold in the glaciers. They feel such a strong desire to sleep, and when their friends try to wake them, warning them of death, they say, "Let me die, I want to sleep." We all cling to the little things of the senses, even if we are ruined thereby; we forget there are much greater things. (8:127)

Every thought that we think, every deed that we do, after a certain time becomes fine, goes into seed form, so to speak, and lives in the fine body in a potential form, and after a time it emerges again and bears its results. These results condition the life of man. Thus he molds his own life. Man is not bound by any other laws excepting those which he makes for himself. Our thoughts, our words and deeds are the threads of the net which we throw round ourselves, for good or for evil. Once we set in motion a certain power, we have to take the full consequences of it. This is the law of karma. (2:348)

Men found out ages ago that the soul is not bound or limited by the senses, no, not even by consciousness. We have to understand that this consciousness is only the name of one link in the infinite chain. Being is not identical with consciousness, but consciousness is only one part of Being. Beyond consciousness is where the bold search lies. Consciousness is bound by the senses. Beyond that, beyond the senses, men must go in order to arrive at truths of the spiritual world, and there are even now persons who succeed in going beyond the bounds of the senses. (3:253)

Method

What makes a man a genius, a sage? Isn't it because he thinks, reasons, wills? Without exercise, the power of deep thinking is lost. Tamas prevails, the mind gets dull and inert, the spirit is brought down to the level of matter. (4:473)

We are responsible for what we are; and whatever we wish ourselves to be, we have the power to make ourselves. If what we are now has been the result of our own past actions, it certainly follows that whatever we wish to be in future can be produced by our present actions; so we have to know how to act. (1:31)

The ideal of all education, all training, should be this man-making. But, instead of that, we are always trying to polish up the outside. What use in polishing up the outside when there is no inside? The end and aim of all training is to make the man grow. The man who influences, who throws his magic, as it were, upon his fellow beings, is a dynamo of power, and when that man is ready, he can do anything and everything he likes; that personality put upon anything will make it work. (2:15)

Moments of grief very often bring out a better spiritual realization. As if for a while the clouds withdraw and the sun of truth shines out. In the case of some, half of the bondage is loosened. Of all bondages the greatest is that of position—the fear of reputation is stronger than the fear of death; but even this bondage appears to relax a little. As if the mind sees for a moment that it is much better to listen to the indwelling Lord than to the opinions of men. But again the clouds close up, and this indeed is maya. (6:392-93)

What avails it if you have power over the whole of the world, if you have mastered every atom in the universe? That will not make you happy unless you have the power of happiness in yourself, until you have conquered yourself. (4:155)

Worship everything as God—every form is His temple. All else is delusion. Always look within, never without. Such is the God that Vedanta preaches, and such is His worship. (8:136)

Above all, follow this great doctrine of sameness in all things, through all beings, seeing the same God in all. (4:328)

True, that spiritual illumination shines of itself in a pure heart, and, as such, it is not something acquired from without; but to attain this purity of heart means long struggle and constant practice. It has also been found, on careful inquiry in the sphere of material knowledge, that those higher truths which have now and then been discovered by great scientific men have flashed like sudden floods of light in their mental atmosphere, which they had only to catch and formulate. But such truths never appear in the mind of an uncultured and wild savage. All these go to prove that hard tapasya, or practice of austerities in the shape of devout contemplation and constant study of a subject, is at the root of all illumination in its respective spheres. (4:436)

Conscious efforts lead the way to superconscious illumination. (4:437)

The Fact of Inner Divinity

The more I live, the more I become convinced every day that every human being is divine. In no man or woman, however vile, does that divinity die. Only he or she does not know how to reach it and is waiting for the Truth. (8:186)

The infinite human soul can never be satisfied but by the Infinite itself. (4:240)

Until we realize God for ourselves, we can know nothing about Him. Each man is perfect by his nature; prophets have manifested this perfection, but it is potential in us. (7:97)

In practical daily life we are hurt by small things; we are enslaved by little beings. Misery comes because we think we are finite—we are little beings. And yet how difficult it is to believe that we are infinite beings! In the midst of all this misery and trouble, when a little thing may throw me off my balance, it must be my care to believe that I am infinite. And the fact is that we are, and that consciously or unconsciously we are all searching after that something which is infinite; we are always seeking for something that is free. (2:399)

Potentially, each one of us has that infinite ocean of Existence, Knowledge, and Bliss as our birthright, our real nature; and the difference between us is caused by the greater or lesser power to manifest that divine. Therefore the Vedanta lays down that each man should be treated not as what he manifests, but as what he stands for. Each human being stands for the divine, and, therefore, every teacher should be helpful, not by condemning man, but by helping him to call forth the divinity that is within him. (1:388)

But the goal of all is the knowledge of the Self, the realization of this Self. To it all men, all beings have equal right. This is the view acceptable to all. (6:457)

In Touch with Perfection

Man is the apex of the only "world" we can ever know. Those who have attained "sameness" or perfection, are said to be "living in God." All hatred is "killing the self by the self"; therefore, love is the law of life. To rise to this is to be perfect. (8:35)

Herein lies the whole secret of existence. Waves may roll over the surface and tempest rage, but deep down there is the stratum of infinite calmness, infinite peace, and infinite bliss. (4:354)

The finite, manifested man forgets his source and thinks himself to be entirely separate. We, as personalized, differentiated beings, forget our reality, and the teaching of monism is not that we shall give up these differentiations, but we must learn to understand what they are. We are in reality that Infinite Being, and our personalities represent so many channels through which this Infinite Reality is manifesting Itself; and the whole mass of changes which we call evolution is brought about by the soul trying to manifest more and more of its infinite energy. We cannot stop anywhere on this side of the Infinite; our power, and blessedness, and wisdom, cannot but grow into the Infinite. Infinite power and existence and blessedness are ours, and we have not to acquire them; they are our own, and we have only to manifest them. (2:339)

What we want is to see the man who is harmoniously developed. . . . We want the man whose heart feels intensely the miseries and sorrows of the world; the man who not only can feel but can find the meaning of things, who delves deeply into the heart of nature and understanding; the man who will not even stop there, who wants to work. Such a combination of head, heart, and hand is what we want. . . . Why not the giant who is equally active, equally knowing, and equally loving? Is it impossible? Certainly not. This is the man of the future, of whom there are few at present. (6:49–50)

Think of this. Compare the great teachers of religion with the great philosophers. The philosophers scarcely influenced anybody's inner man, and yet they wrote most marvelous books. The religious teachers, on the other hand, moved countries in their lifetime. The difference was made by personality. In the philosopher it is a faint personality that influences; in the great prophets it is tremendous. In the former we touch the intellect, in the latter we touch life. (2:15)

The knowledge of man is the highest knowledge, and only by knowing man can we know God. This is also a fact, that the knowledge of God is the highest knowledge, and knowing God alone we can know man. Apparently contradictory though these statements may appear, they are the necessity of human nature. (1:433)

7

SOBERING THE MONKEY

The Mind in Action

How hard it is to control the mind! Well has it been compared to the maddened monkey. There was a monkey, restless by his own nature, as all monkeys are. As if that were not enough, someone made him drink freely of wine, so that he became still more restless. Then a scorpion stung him. When a man is stung by a scorpion, he jumps about for a whole day; so the poor monkey found his condition worse than ever. To complete his misery, a demon entered into him. What language can describe the uncontrollable restlessness of that monkey? The human mind is like that monkey, incessantly active by its own nature; then it becomes drunk with the wine of desire, thus increasing its turbulence. After desire takes possession comes the sting of the scorpion of jealousy at the success of others, and last of all the demon of pride enters the mind, making it think itself of all importance. How hard to control such a mind! (1:174)

All knowledge that the world has ever received comes from the mind; the infinite library of the universe is in your own mind. (1:28)

Nature is the quality of the plant, the quality of the animal, and the quality of man. Man's life behaves according to definite methods; so does his mind. Thoughts do not just happen, there is a certain method in their rise, existence, and fall. In other words, just as external phenomena are bound by law, internal phenomena, that is to say, the life and mind of man, are also bound by law. (8:244)

This mind is like a lake, and every thought is like a wave upon that lake. Just as the lake-waves rise and then fall down and disappear, so these thought-waves are continually rising in the mind-stuff and then disappearing, but they do not disappear forever. They become finer and finer, but they are all there, ready to start up at another time when called upon to do so. Memory is simply calling back into wave-form some of those thoughts which have gone into that finer state of existence. Thus, everything that we have thought, every action that we have done, is lodged in the mind; it is all there in fine form, and when a man dies, the sum total of these impressions is in the mind, which again works upon a little fine material as a medium. The soul, clothed, as it were, with these impressions and the fine body, passes out, and the destiny of the soul is guided by the resultant of all the different forces represented by the different impressions. (2:268–69)

Meditation has been laid stress upon by all religions. The meditative state of mind is declared by the yogis to be the highest state in which the mind exists. When the mind is studying the external object, it gets identified with it, loses itself. To use the simile of the old Indian philosopher: the soul of man is like a piece of crystal, but it takes the color of whatever is near it. Whatever the soul touches . . . it has to take its color. That is the difficulty. That constitutes the bondage. The color is so strong, the crystal forgets itself and identifies itself with the color. Suppose a red flower is near the crystal: the crystal takes the color and forgets itself, thinks it is red. We have taken the color of the body and have forgotten what we are. All the difficulties that follow come from that one dead body. All our fears, all worries, anxieties, troubles, mistakes, weakness, evil, are from that one great blunder—that we are bodies. This is the ordinary person. It is the person taking the color of the flower near to it. We are no more bodies than the crystal is the red flower. (4:227)

Turning the Mind Within

From our childhood upward we have been taught only to pay attention to things external, but never to things internal; hence most of us have nearly lost the faculty of observing the internal mechanism. To turn the mind, as it were, inside, stop it from going outside, and then to concentrate all its powers, and throw them upon the mind itself, in order that it may know its own nature, analyze itself, is very hard work. Yet that is the only way to anything which will be a scientific approach to the subject. (1:129–30)

It is good and very grand to conquer external nature, but grander still to conquer our internal nature. It is grand and good to know the laws that govern the stars and planets; it is infinitely grander and better to know the laws that govern the passions, the feelings, the will of mankind. This conquering of the inner man, understanding the secrets of the subtle workings that are within the human mind, and knowing its wonderful secrets, belong entirely to religion. (2:65)

The mind has to be gradually and systematically brought under control. The will has to be strengthened by slow, continuous, and persevering drill. This is no child's play, no fad to be tried one day and discarded the next. It is a life's work; and the end to be attained is well worth all that it can cost us to reach it; being nothing less than the realization of our absolute oneness with the Divine. Surely, with this end in view, and with the knowledge that we can certainly succeed, no price can be too great to pay. (5:294)

The purer the mind, the easier it is to control it. (4:220)

How has all the knowledge in the world been gained but by the concentration of the powers of the mind? The world is ready to give up its secrets if we only know how to knock, how to give it the necessary blow. The strength and force of the blow come through concentration. There is no limit to the power of the human mind.

The more concentrated it is, the more power is brought to bear on one point; that is the secret.

It is easy to concentrate the mind on external things, the mind naturally goes outward; but not so in the case of religion, or psychology, or metaphysics, where the subject and the object are one. The object is internal, the mind itself is the object, and it is necessary to study the mind itself—mind studying mind. We know that there is the power of the mind called reflection. I am talking to you. At the same time I am standing aside, as it were, a second person, and knowing and hearing what I am talking. You work and think at the same time, while a portion of your mind stands by and sees what you are thinking. The powers of the mind should be concentrated and turned back upon itself, and as the darkest places reveal their secrets before the penetrating rays of the sun, so will this concentrated mind penetrate its own innermost secrets. Thus will we come to the basis of belief, the real genuine religion. We will perceive for ourselves whether we have souls, whether life is of five minutes or of eternity, whether there is a God in the universe or more. It will all be revealed to us. (1:130–31)

The mind-waves, which are gross, we can appreciate and feel, they can be more easily controlled; but what about the finer instincts? How can they be controlled? When I am angry, my whole mind becomes a huge wave of anger. I feel it, see it, handle it, can easily manipulate it, can fight with it; but I shall not succeed perfectly in the fight until I can get down below to its causes. A man says something very harsh to me, and I begin to feel that I am getting heated, and he goes on till I am perfectly angry and forget myself, identify myself with anger. When he first began to abuse me, I thought, "I am going to be angry." Anger was one thing, and I was another; but when I became angry, I was anger. These feelings have to be controlled in the germ, the root, in their fine forms, before even we have become conscious that they are acting on us. With the vast majority of mankind the fine states of these passions are not even known—the states in which they emerge from subconsciousness. When a bubble is rising from the bottom of the lake, we do not see it, nor even when it is nearly come to the surface; it is only when it bursts and makes a ripple that we know it is there. We shall only be successful in grappling with the waves when we can get hold of them in their fine causes, and until you can get hold of them, and subdue them before they become gross, there is no hope of conquering any passion perfectly. To control our passions we have to control them at their very roots; then alone shall we be able to burn out their very seeds. As fried seeds thrown into the ground will never come up, so these passions will never arise. (1:241–42)

Every vicious thought will rebound, every thought of hatred which you may have thought, in a cave even, is stored up, and will one day come back to you with tremendous power in the form of some misery here. If you project hatred and jealousy, they will rebound on you with compound interest. (1:262)

The disciple must have great power of endurance. Life seems comfortable; and you find the mind behaves well when everything is going well with you. But if something goes wrong, your mind loses its balance. That is not good. Bear all evil and misery without one murmur of hurt, without one thought of unhappiness, resistance, remedy, or retaliation. That is true endurance; and that you must acquire. (8:110)

The reason why a criminal is a criminal is not because he desires to be one, but because he does not have his mind under control and is therefore a slave to his own conscious and subconscious mind, and to the minds of everybody else. (6:29)

Hold to the idea, "I am not the mind, I see that I am thinking, I am watching my mind act," and each day the identification of yourself with thought and feeling will grow less, until at last you can entirely separate yourself from the mind and actually know it to be apart from yourself.

When this is done, the mind is your servant to control as you will. The first stage of being a yogi is to go beyond the senses. When the mind is conquered, he has reached the highest stage. (8:48)

The Concentrated Mind

How are we to know that the mind has become concentrated? Because the idea of time will vanish. The more time passes unnoticed, the more concentrated we are. In common life we see that when we are interested in a book we do not note the time at all; and when we leave the book, we are often surprised to find how many hours have passed. All time will have the tendency to come and stand in the one present. So the definition is given: When the past and present come and stand in one, the mind is said to be concentrated. (1:273–74)

This meditative state is the highest state of existence. So long as there is desire, no real happiness can come. It is only the contemplative, witnesslike study of objects that brings to us real enjoyment and happiness. The animal has its happiness in the senses, the man in his intellect, and the god in spiritual contemplation. It is only to the soul that has attained to this contemplative state that the world really becomes beautiful. To him who desires nothing, and does not mix himself up with them, the manifold changes of nature are one panorama of beauty and sublimity. (1:186–87)

When by analyzing his own mind, man comes face to face, as it were, with something which is never destroyed, something which is, by its own nature, eternally pure and perfect, he will no more be miserable, no more unhappy. All misery comes from fear, from unsatisfied desire. Man will find that he never dies, and then he will have no more fear of death. When he knows that he is perfect, he will have no more vain desires, and both these causes being absent, there will be no more misery—there will be perfect bliss, even while in this body. (1:130)

Some say that by controlling internal nature we control everything. Others that by controlling external nature we control everything. Carried to the extreme both are right, because in nature
there is no such division as internal or external. These are fictitious
limitations that never existed. The externalists and the internalists
are destined to meet at the same point, when both reach the
extreme of their knowledge. Just as a physicist, when he pushes his
knowledge to its limits, finds it melting away into metaphysics, so
a metaphysician will find that what he calls mind and matter are
but apparent distinctions, the reality being One. (1:133)

Each time we suppress hatred, or a feeling of anger, it is so much
good energy stored up in our favor; that piece of energy will be
converted into the higher powers. (1:223)

When the imagination is very powerful, the object becomes
visualized. Therefore by it we can bring our bodies to any state of
health or disease. When we see a thing, the particles of the brain
fall into a certain position like the mosaics of a kaleidoscope.
Memory consists in getting back this combination and the same
setting of the particles of the brain. The stronger the will, the
greater will be the success in resetting these particles of the brain.
There is only one power to cure the body, and that is in every man.
Medicine only rouses this power. Disease is only the manifest
struggle of that power to throw off the posion which has entered
the body. Although the power to overthrow poison may be roused
by medicine, it may be more permanently roused by the force of
thought. Imagination must hold to the thought of health and
strength in order that in case of illness the memory of the ideal of
health may be roused and the particles rearranged in the position
into which they fell when healthy. The tendency of the body is then
to follow the brain. (6:133–34)

When the yogi has attained to discrimination, all powers come
to him, but the true yogi rejects them all. Unto him comes a
peculiar knowledge, a particular light, called the dharma-megha,

the cloud of virtue. All the great prophets of the world, whom history has recorded, had this. They had found the whole foundation of knowledge within themselves. Truth to them had become real. Peace and calmness, and perfect purity became their own nature, after they had given up the vanities of power. (1:302)

8

WORK AS SELF-TRANSFORMATION

Doing Good to Others

The more intently you think of the well-being of others, the more oblivious of self you become. In this way, as gradually your heart gets purified by work, you will come to feel the truth that your own Self is pervading all beings and all things. Thus it is that doing good to others constitutes a way, a means of revealing one's own Self or Atman. Know this also to be one of the spiritual practices, a discipline for God-realization. (7:112)

Charity is great, but the moment you say it is all, you run the risk of running into materialism. (4:239)

That purity which is the goal of work is realizable only through doing good to others. (6:311)

Oh, how calm would be the work of one who really understood the divinity of man! For such, there is nothing to do, save to open men's eyes. All the rest does itself. (8:261)

The essential thing is renunciation. Without renunciation none can pour out his whole heart in working for others. The man of renunciation sees all with an equal eye and devotes himself to the service of all. (5:382)

Look upon every man, woman, and everyone as God. You cannot help anyone, you can only serve: serve the children of the Lord, serve the Lord Himself, if you have the privilege. If the Lord grants that you can help any one of His children, blessed you are; do not think too much of yourselves. Blessed you are that that privilege was given to you when others had it not. Do it only as a worship. I should see God in the poor, and it is for my salvation that I go and worship them. The poor and the miserable are for our salvation, so that we may serve the Lord, coming in the shape of the diseased, coming in the shape of the lunatic, the leper, and the sinner! Bold are my words; and let me repeat that it is the greatest privilege in our life that we are allowed to serve the Lord in all these shapes. Give up the idea that by ruling over others you can do any good to them. (3:246–47)

Bring all light into the world. Light, bring light! Let light come unto everyone; the task will not be finished till everyone has reached the Lord. Bring light to the poor; and bring more light to the rich, for they require it more than the poor. Bring light to the ignorant, and more light to the educated, for the vanities of the educated of our time are tremendous! Thus bring light to all and leave the rest unto the Lord, for in the words of the same Lord, "To work you have the right and not to the fruits thereof." "Let not your work produce results for *you*, and at the same time may you never be without work." (3:247)

Thank God for giving you this world as a moral gymnasium to help your development, but never imagine you can help the world. (7:69)

Ends and Means

One of the greatest lessons I have learnt in my life is to pay as much attention to the means of work as to its end. (2:1)

Work and worship are necessary to take away the veil, to lift off the bondage and illusion. They do not give us freedom; but all the same, without effort on our own part we do not open our eyes and see what we are. (7:53)

Doing work is not religion, but work done rightly leads to freedom. (7:69)

Proper attention to the finishing, strengthening, of the means is what we need. With the means all right, the end must come. We forget that it is the cause that produces the effect; the effect cannot come by itself; and unless the causes are exact, proper, and powerful, the effect will not be produced. Once the ideal is chosen and the means determined, we may almost let go the ideal, because we are sure it will be there, when the means are perfected. (2:1)

If you set to work in right earnest, then you are sure to be successful. Whoever works at a thing heart and soul not only achieves success in it, but through his absorption in that he also realizes the supreme Truth—Brahman. Whoever works at a thing with his whole heart receives help from God. (7:202)

If you really want to judge the character of a man, look not at his great performances. Every fool may become a hero at one time or another. Watch a man do his most common actions; these are indeed the things which will tell you the real character of a great man. (1:29)

Let Us Go to Work

Whenever mankind attains a higher vision, the lower vision disappears of itself. Multitude counts for nothing. A few heart-whole, sincere, and energetic men can do more in a year than a mob in a century. If there is heat in one body, then those others that come near it must catch it. This is the law. So success is ours, so long as we keep up the heat, the spirit of truth, sincerity, and love. (8:346)

Even the greatest fool can accomplish a task if it be after his heart. But the intelligent man is he who can convert every work into one that suits his taste. No work is petty. Everything in this world is like a banyan seed, which, though appearing tiny as a mustard seed, has yet the gigantic banyan tree latent within it. He indeed is intelligent who notices this and succeeds in making all work truly great. (7:508)

He who grumbles at the little thing that has fallen to his lot to do will grumble at everything. Always grumbling, he will lead a miserable life, and everything will be a failure. But that man who does his duty as he goes, putting his shoulder to the wheel, will see the light, and higher and higher duties will fall to his share. (5:242)

Each work has to pass through these stages—ridicule, opposition, and then acceptance. Each man who thinks ahead of his time is sure to be misunderstood. So opposition and persecution are welcome, only I have to be steady and pure and must have immense faith in God, and all these will vanish. (5:91)

Do any deserve liberty who are not ready to give it to others? Let us calmly and in a manly fashion go to work, instead of dissipating our energy in unnecessary frettings and fumings. I, for one, thoroughly believe that no power in the universe can withhold from anyone anything he really deserves. The past was great no doubt, but I sincerely believe that the future will be more glorious still. (4:366)

Sowing and Reaping

We reap what we sow. We are the makers of our own fate. None else has the blame, none has the praise. (2:224)

Any work, any action, any thought that produces an effect is called a karma. Thus the law of karma means the law of causation, of inevitable cause and sequence. Wheresoever there is a cause, there an effect must be produced; this necessity cannot be resisted, and this law of karma, according to our philosophy, is true throughout the whole universe. Whatever we see, or feel, or do, whatever action there is anywhere in the universe, while being the effect of past work on the one hand, becomes, on the other, a cause in its turn, and produces its own effect. (1:94)

That way, which your nature makes it absolutely necessary for you to take, is the right way. Each one of us is born with a peculiarity of nature as the result of our past existence. Either we call it our own reincarnated past experience or a hereditary past; whatever way we may put it, we are the result of the past—that is absolutely certain, through whatever channels that past may have come. It naturally follows that each one of us in an effect, of which our past has been the cause; and as such, there is a peculiar movement, a peculiar train, in each one of us; and therefore each one will have to find the way for himself. (4:52)

We came to enjoy; we are being enjoyed. We came to rule; we are being ruled. We came to work; we are being worked. All the time, we find that. And this comes into every detail of our life. We are being worked upon by other minds, and we are always struggling to work on other minds. We want to enjoy the pleasures of life; and they eat into our vitals. We want to get everything from nature, but we find in the long run that nature takes everything from us—depletes us, and casts us aside. (2:2)

When we come to nonattachment, then we can understand the marvelous mystery of the universe; how it is intense activity and vibration, and at the same time intensest peace and calm; how it is work every moment and rest every moment. That is the mystery of the universe—the impersonal and personal in one, the infinite and finite in one. (1:442)

Will

Are great things ever done smoothly? Time, patience, and indomitable will must show. (5:93)

What work do you expect from men of little hearts? —Nothing in the world! You must have an iron will if you would cross the ocean. You must be strong enough to pierce mountains. (6:297)

Have you got the will to surmount mountain-high obstructions? If the whole world stands against you sword in hand, would you still dare to do what you think is right? (3:226)

Duty

By doing well the duty which is nearest to us, the duty which is in our hands now, we make ourselves stronger, and improving our strength in this manner step by step, we may even reach a state in which it shall be our privilege to do the most coveted and honored duties in life and in society. (5:240)

Any action that makes us go Godward is a good action, and is our duty; any action that makes us go downward is evil, and is not our duty. From the subjective standpoint we may see that certain acts have a tendency to exalt and ennoble us, while certain other acts have a tendency to degrade and to brutalize us. But it is not possible to make out with certainty which acts have which kind of tendency in relation to all persons, of all sorts and conditions. There is, however, only one idea of duty which has been universally accepted by all mankind, of all ages and sects and countries, and that has been summed up in a Sanskrit aphorism thus: "Do not injure any being; not injuring any being is virtue, injuring any being is sin." (1:64)

Art of Work

He who knows how to obey knows how to command. Learn obedience first. Among the Western nations, with such a high spirit of independence, the spirit of obedience is equally strong. (6:349)

Work on with the intrepidity of a lion, but at the same time with the tenderness of a flower. (6:332)

The less passion there is, the better we work. The calmer we are, the better for us, and the more the amount of work we can do. When we let loose our feelings, we waste so much energy, shatter our nerves, disturb our minds, and accomplish very little work. . . . It is only when the mind is very calm and collected that the whole of its energy is spent in doing good work. And if you read the lives of the great workers which the world has produced, you will find that they were wonderfully calm men. (2:293)

A man should not be judged by the nature of his duties, but by the manner in which he does them. . . . A shoemaker who can turn out a strong, nice pair of shoes in the shortest possible time is a better man, according to his profession and his work, then a professor who talks nonsense every day of his life. (5:239-40)

Skillful management lies in giving every man work after his own heart. (8:455)

Neither seek nor avoid; take what comes. It is liberty to be affected by nothing; do not merely endure, be unattached. Remember the story of the bull. A mosquito sat long on the horn of a certain bull. Then his conscience troubled him, and he said, "Mr. Bull, I have been sitting here a long time, perhaps I annoy you. I am sorry, I will go away." But the bull replied, "Oh no, not at all! Bring your whole family and live on my horn; what can you do to me?" (7:14)

Those who work without any consciousness of their lower ego are not affected with evil, for they work for the good of the world. To work without motive, to work unattached, brings the highest bliss and freedom. (5:249)

Just as water cannot wet the lotus leaf, so work cannot bind the unselfish man by giving rise to attachment to results. The selfless and unattached man may live in the very heart of a crowded and sinful city; he will not be touched by sin. (1:60)

You are the soul, the pure, the free, all the time; you are the Witness. Our misery comes, not from work, but by our getting attached to something. Take for instance, money: money is a great thing to have, earn it, says Krishna; struggle hard to get money, but don't get attached to it. So with children, with wife, husband, relatives, fame, everything; you have no need to shun them, only don't get attached. There is only one attachment and that belongs to the Lord, and to none other. Work for them, love them, do good to them, sacrifice a hundred lives, if need be, for them, but never be attached. (4:96)

Everything that you do under compulsion goes to build up attachment. Why should you have any duty? Resign everything unto God. In this tremendous fiery furnace where the fire of duty scorches everybody, drink this cup of nectar and be happy. We are all simply working out His will, and have nothing to do with rewards and punishments. If you want the reward, you must also have the punishment; the only way to get out of the punishment is to give up the reward. The only way of getting out of misery is by giving up the idea of happiness, because these two are linked to each other. On one side there is happiness, on the other there is misery. On one side there is life, on the other there is death. The only way to get beyond death is to give up the love of life. Life and death are the same thing, looked at from different points. So the idea of happiness without misery, or of life without death, is very good for schoolboys and children; but the thinker sees that it is all a contradiction in terms and gives up both. (1:104)

Great Works

No one ever succeeded in keeping society in good humor and at the same time did great works. One must work as the dictate comes from within, and then if it is right and good, society is bound to veer round, perhaps centuries after one is dead and gone. We must plunge heart and soul and body into the work. (6:301)

Purity, patience, and perseverance are the three essentials to success and, above all, *love*. (6:281)

Was it ever in the history of the world that any great work was done by the rich? It is the heart and the brain that do it ever and ever and not the purse. (6:302)

9

TRAINING THE MIND
FOR WISDOM

First Steps

We are to take care of ourselves—that much we can do—and give up attending to others for a time. Let us perfect the means; the end will take care of itself. For the world can be good and pure, only if our lives are good and pure. It is an effect, and we are the means. Therefore, let us purify ourselves. Let us make ourselves perfect. (2:9)

Duty is seldom sweet. It is only when love greases its wheels that it runs smoothly; it is a continuous friction otherwise. (1:67)

He who wants to enter the realms of light must make a bundle of all "shopkeeping" religion and cast it away before he can pass the gates. It is not that you do not get what you pray for; you get everything, but it is low, vulgar, a beggar's religion. (7:83–84)

Believe, therefore, in yourselves, and if you want material wealth, work it out; it will come to you. If you want to be intellectual, work it out on the intellectual plane, and intellectual giants you shall be. And if you want to attain to freedom, work it out on the spiritual plane, and free you shall be. (3:427)

He who always speculates as to what awaits him in the future, accomplishes nothing whatsoever. What you have understood as true and good, just do that at once. What's the good of calculating what may or may not befall in the future? The span of life is so, so short—and can anything be accomplished in it if you go on forecasting and computing results? God is the only dispenser of results; leave it to Him to do all that. What have you got to do with it? Don't look that way, but go on working. (6:455)

We must not be extremely attached to anything excepting God. See everything, do everything, but be not attached. As soon as extreme attachment comes, a man loses himself, he is no more master of himself, he is a slave. If a woman is tremendously attached to a man, she becomes a slave to that man. There is no use in being a slave. There are higher things in this world than becoming a slave to a human being. Love and do good to everybody, but do not become a slave. In the first place, attachment degenerates us individually, and in the second place, makes us extremely selfish. Owing to this failing, we want to injure others to do good to those we love. A good many of the wicked deeds done in this world are really done through attachment to certain persons. So all attachment excepting that for good works should be avoided; but love should be given to everybody. (4:6)

A man used to solitude, if brought in contact with the surging whirlpool of the world, will be crushed by it; just as the fish that lives in the deep sea water, as soon as it is brought to the surface, breaks into pieces, deprived of the weight of water on it that had kept it together. Can a man who has been used to the turmoil and the rush of life live at ease if he comes to a quiet place? He suffers and perchance may lose his mind. The ideal man is he who, in the midst of the greatest silence and solitude, finds the intensest activity, and in the midst of the intensest activity finds the silence and solitude of the desert. (1:34)

Always keep your mind joyful; if melancholy thoughts come, kick them out. (6:130)

[Will not the spirit break down at the thought of death and the heart be overpowered by despondency?] Quite so. At first, the heart will break down, and despondency and gloomy thoughts will occupy your mind. But persist, let days pass like that—and then? Then you will see that new strength has come into the heart, that the constant thought of death is giving you a new life and is making you more and more thoughtful. (5:329)

Isolation of the soul from all objects, mental and physical, is the goal; when that is attained, the soul will find that it was alone all the time, and it required no one to make it happy. As long as we require someone else to make us happy, we are slaves. (5:239)

Do not pity anyone. Look upon all as your equal, cleanse yourself of the primal sin of inequality. We are all equal and must not think, "I am good and you are bad, and I am trying to reclaim you." Equality is the sign of the free. (8:18)

Thought, the Propelling Force

It is thought which is the propelling force in us. Fill the mind with the highest thoughts, hear them day after day, think them month after month. Never mind failures; they are quite natural, they are the beauty of life, these failures. What would life be without them? It would not be worth having if it were not for struggles. Where would be the poetry of life? Never mind the struggles, the mistakes. I never heard a cow tell a lie, but it is only a cow—never a man. So never mind these failures, these little backslidings; hold the ideal a thousand times, and if you fail a thousand times, make the attempt once more. The ideal of man is to see God in everything. But if you cannot see Him in everything, see Him in one thing, in that thing which you like best, and then see Him in another. So on you can go. There is infinite life before the soul. Take your time, and you will achieve your end. (2:152–53)

Whatever you dream and think of, you create. If it is hell, you die and see hell. If it is evil and Satan, you get Satan. If ghosts, you get ghosts. Whatever you think, that you become. If you have to think, think good thoughts, great thoughts. This taking for granted that you are weak little worms! By declaring we are weak, we become weak, we do not become better. Suppose we put out the light, close the windows, and call the room dark. Think of the nonsense! What good does it do me to say I am a sinner? If I am in the dark, let me light a lamp. (8:130–31)

In this universe where nothing is lost, where we live in the midst of death *in life*, every thought that is thought, in public or in private, in crowded thoroughfares or in the deep recesses of primeval forests, lives. They are continuously trying to become self-embodied, and until they have embodied themselves, they will struggle for expression, and any amount of repression cannot kill them. Nothing can be destroyed—those thoughts that caused evil in the past are also seeking embodiment, to be filtered through repeated expression and, at last, transfigured into perfect good. (6:354)

Body is only mind in a grosser form, mind being composed of finer layers and the body being the denser layers; and when man has perfect control over his mind, he will also have control over his body. (6:140–41)

Unfortunately in this life the vast majority of persons are groping through this dark life without any ideal at all. If a man with an ideal makes a thousand mistakes, I am sure that the man without an ideal makes fifty thousand. Therefore, it is better to have an ideal. And this ideal we must hear about as much as we can, till it enters into our hearts, into our brains, into our very veins, until it tingles in every drop of our blood and permeates every pore in our body. We must meditate upon it. (2:152)

Few understand the power of thought. If a man goes into a cave, shuts himself in, and thinks one really great thought and dies, that thought will penetrate the walls of that cave, vibrate through space, and at last permeate the whole human race. Such is the power of thought; be in no hurry therefore to give your thoughts to others. First have something to give. He alone teaches who has something to give, for teaching is not talking, teaching is not imparting doctrines, it is communicating. Spirituality can be communicated just as really as I can give you a flower. This is true in the most literal sense. (4:177–78)

Behind the Veil of Appearances

The misery that we suffer comes from ignorance, from nondiscrimination between the real and the unreal. We all take the bad for the good, the dream for the reality. Soul is the only reality, and we have forgotten it. Body is an unreal dream, and we think we are all bodies. This nondiscrimination is the cause of misery. It is caused by ignorance. When discrimination comes, it brings strength, and then alone can we avoid all these various ideas of body, heavens, and gods. (1:287)

If you know that you are positively other than your body, you have then none to fight with or struggle against; you are dead to all ideas of selfishness. (3:84)

The mind brings before us all our delusions—body, sex, creed, caste, bondage; so we have to tell the truth to the mind incessantly, until it is made to realize it. Our real nature is all bliss, and all the pleasure we know is but a reflection, an atom, of that bliss we get from touching our real nature. (8:7)

The present is only a line of demarcation between the past and the future; so we cannot rationally say that we care only for the present, as it has no existence apart from the past and the future. It is all one complete whole, the idea of time being merely a condition imposed upon us by the form of our understanding. (8:9)

There is really no difference between matter, mind, and Spirit. They are only different phases of experiencing the One. This very world is seen by the five senses as matter, by the very wicked as hell, by the good as heaven, and by the perfect as God. (5:272)

That is the highest when the subject and the object become one. When I am the listener and I am the speaker, when I am the teacher and I am the taught, when I am the creator and I am the created—then alone fear ceases; there is not another to make us afraid. There is nothing but myself, what can frighten me? This is to be heard day after day. Get rid of all other thoughts. Everything else must be thrown aside, and this is to be repeated continually, poured through the ears until it reaches the heart, until every nerve and muscle, every drop of blood tingles with the idea that I am He, I am He. Even at the gate of death say, "I am He." (3:25–26)

When we have given up desires, then alone shall we be able to read and enjoy this universe of God. Then everything will become deified. Nooks and corners, by-ways and shady places, which we thought dark and unholy, will be all deified. They will all reveal their true nature, and we shall smile at ourselves and think that all this weeping and crying has been but child's play, and we were only standing by, watching.

So, do your work, says the Vedanta. It first advises us how to work—by giving up—giving up the apparent, illusive world. What is meant by that? Seeing God everywhere. Thus do your work. (2:149)

Getting Out of the Old Groove

Only the fools rush after sense-enjoyments. It is easy to live in the senses. It is easier to run in the old groove, eating and drinking; but what these modern philosophers want to tell you is to take these comfortable ideas and put the stamp of religion on them. Such a doctrine is dangerous. Death lies in the senses. Life on the plane of the Spirit is the only life, life on any other plane is mere death; the whole of this life can be only described as a gymnasium. We must go beyond it to enjoy real life. (5:267)

The ideal is really that we should become many-sided. Indeed the cause of the misery of the world is that we are so one-sided that we cannot sympathize with one another. Consider a man looking at the sun from beneath the earth, up the shaft of a mine; he sees one aspect of the sun. Then another man sees the sun from the earth's level, another through mist and fog, another from the mountain top. To each the sun has a different appearance. So there are many appearances, but in reality there is only one sun. There is diversity of vision, but one object; and that is the sun. (6:137)

You keep this body as long as you like. If you do not like it, do not have it. The Infinite is the real; the finite is the play. (2:471)

The first thing to be got rid of by him who would be a jnani is fear. Fear is one of our worst enemies. Next, believe in nothing until you *know* it. Constantly tell yourself, "I am not the body, I am not the mind, I am not thought, I am not even consciousness; I am the Atman." When you can throw away *all*, only the true Self will remain. (8:4)

We shall all die! Bear this in mind always, and then the spirit within will wake up. (5:329)

Truth, Reason, and Inspiration

Think for yourself. No blind belief can save you, work out your own salvation. (7:86)

Is it not tremendously blasphemous to believe against reason? What right have we not to use the greatest gift that God has given to us? I am sure God will pardon a man who will use his reason and cannot believe, rather than a man who believes blindly instead of using the faculties He has given him. (6:12–13)

Inspiration is much higher than reason, but it must not contradict it. Reason is the rough tool to do the hard work; inspiration is the bright light which shows us all truth. The will to do a thing is not necessarily inspiration. (7:91–92)

Human knowledge is not antagonistic to human well-being. On the contrary, it is knowledge alone that will save us in every department of life—in knowledge is worship. The more we know the better for us. (2:355)

I will compare truth to a corrosive substance of infinite power. It burns its way in wherever it falls—in soft substance at once, hard granite slowly, but it must. (5:71)

To get any reason out of the mass of incongruity we call human life, we have to transcend our reason, but we must do it scientifically, slowly, by regular practice, and we must cast off all superstition. We must take up the study of the superconscious state just as any other science. On reason we must have to lay our foundation, we must follow reason as far as it leads, and when reason fails, reason itself will show us the way to the highest plane. When you hear a man say, "I am inspired," and then talk irrationally, reject it. Why? Because these three states—instinct, reason, and super-consciousness, or the unconscious, conscious, and superconscious states—belong to one and the same mind. There are not three minds in one man, but one state of it develops into others. Instinct develops into reason and reason into the transcendental consciousness; therefore, not one of the states contradicts the others. Real inspiration never contradicts reason, but fulfills it. Just as you find the great prophets saying, "I come not to destroy but to fulfill," so inspiration always comes to fulfill reason, and is in harmony with it. (1:184–85)

Great truths are simple because they are of universal application. Truth itself is always simple. Complexity is due to man's ignorance. (6:35)

"Comfort" is no test of truth; on the contrary, truth is often far from being "comfortable." If one intends to really find truth, one must not cling to comfort. It is hard to let all go, but the jnani *must* do it. He must become pure, kill out all desires and cease to identify himself with the body. Then and then only, the higher truth can shine in his soul. (8:14)

Realization is real religion, all the rest is only preparation—hearing lectures, or reading books, or reasoning is merely preparing the ground; it is not religion. Intellectual assent and intellectual dissent are not religion. The central idea of the yogis is that just as we come in direct contact with objects of the senses, so religion even can be directly perceived in a far more intense sense. (1:232)

Is religion to justify itself by the discoveries of reason, through which every other science justifies itself? Are the same methods of investigation, which we apply to sciences and knowledge outside, to be applied to the science of religion? In my opinion this must be so, and I am also of opinion that the sooner it is done the better. If a religion is destroyed by such investigations, it was then all the time useless, unworthy superstition; and the sooner it goes the better. I am thoroughly convinced that its destruction would be the best thing that could happen. All that is dross will be taken off, no doubt, but the essential parts of religion will emerge triumphant out of this investigation. Not only will it be made scientific—as scientific, at least, as any of the conclusions of physics or chemistry—but will have greater strength, because physics or chemistry has no internal mandate to vouch for its truth, which religion has. (1:367)

When there is conflict between the heart and the brain, let the heart be followed, because intellect has only one state, reason, and within that, intellect works, and cannot get beyond. It is the heart which takes one to the highest plane, which intellect can never reach; it goes beyond intellect, and reaches to what is called inspiration. (1:412–13)

Avoiding Spiritual Decay

Raja yoga does not, after the unpardonable manner of some modern scientists, deny the existence of facts which are difficult to explain; on the other hand, it gently, yet in no uncertain terms, tells the superstitious that miracles, and answers to prayers, and powers of faith, though true as facts, are not rendered comprehensible through the superstitious explanation of attributing them to the agency of a being, or beings, above the clouds. It declares that each man is only a conduit for the infinite ocean of knowledge and power that lies behind mankind. It teaches that desires and wants are in man, that the power of supply is also in man; and that wherever and whenever a desire, a want, a prayer has been fulfilled, it was out of this infinite magazine that the supply came, and not from any supernatural being. The idea of supernatural beings may rouse to a certain extent the power of action in man, but it also brings spiritual decay. It brings dependence; it brings fear; it brings superstition. It degenerates into a horrible belief in the natural weakness of man. There is no supernatural, says the yogi, but there are in nature gross manifestations and subtle manifestations. The subtle are the causes, the gross the effects. The gross can be easily perceived by the senses; not so the subtle. (1:121–22)

Anything that is secret and mysterious in these systems of yoga should be at once rejected. The best guide in life is strength. In religion, as in all other matters, discard everything that weakens you, have nothing to do with it. (1:134)

The great danger of psychic powers is that man stumbles, as it were, into them, and knows not how to use them rightly. He is without training and without knowledge of what has happened to him. The danger is that in using these psychic powers, the sexual feelings are abnormally roused as these powers are in fact manufactured out of the sexual center. (6:131)

All these secret societies and humbugs make men and women impure, weak, and narrow; and the weak have no will, and can never work. Therefore have nothing to do with them. All this false love of mystery should be knocked on the head the first time it comes into your mind. No one who is the least impure will ever become religious. Do not try to cover festering sores with masses of roses. Do you think you can cheat God? None can. Give me a straightforward man or woman; but Lord save me from ghosts, flying angels, and devils. Be common, everyday, nice people. (4:58)

The Ways of the Wise

Two ways are left open to us—the way of the ignorant, who think that there is only one way to truth and that all the rest are wrong, and the way of the wise, who admit that, according to our mental constitution or the different planes of existence in which we are, duty and morality may vary. The important thing is to know that there are gradations of duty and of morality—that the duty of one state of life, in one set of circumstances, will not and cannot be that of another.

To illustrate: All great teachers have taught, "Resist not evil," that nonresistance is the highest moral ideal. We all know that, if a certain number of us attempted to put that maxim fully into practice, the whole social fabric would fall to pieces, the wicked would take possession of our properties and our lives, and would do whatever they liked with us. Even if only one day of such nonresistance were practiced, it would lead to disaster. Yet, intuitively, in our heart of hearts we feel the truth of the teaching "Resist not evil." This seems to us to be the highest ideal; yet to teach this doctrine only would be equivalent to condemning a vast portion of mankind. Not only so, it would be making men feel that they were always doing wrong, and cause in them scruples of conscious in all their actions; it would weaken them, and that constant self-disapproval would breed more vice than any other weakness would. To the man who has begun to hate himself the gate to degeneration has already opened; and the same is true of a nation. (1:37–38)

We only get what we deserve. It is a lie when we say the world is bad and we are good. It can never be so. It is a terrible lie we tell ourselves.

This is the first lesson to learn: be determined not to curse anything outside, not to lay the blame upon anyone outside, but be a man, stand up, lay the blame on yourself. You will find that is always true. Get hold of yourself. (2:8)

Spiritual knowledge is the only thing that can destroy our miseries forever; any other knowledge satisfies wants only for a time. (1:52)

Often and often we see that the very best of men even are troubled and visited with tribulations in this world; it may be inexplicable; but it is also the experience of my life that the heart and core of everything here is good, that whatever may be the surface waves, deep down and underlying everything, there is an infinite basis of goodness and love; and so long as we do not reach that basis, we are troubled; but having once reached that zone of calmness, let winds howl and tempests rage. (8:296)

The only test of good things is that they make us strong. (8:185)

It is remarkable that almost every good idea in this world can be carried to a disgusting extreme. (3:67)

There is no progress in a straight line. Every soul moves in a circle, as it were, and will have to complete it; and no soul can go so low but that there will come a time when it will have to go upward. It may start straight down, but it has to take the upward curve to complete the circuit. We are all projected from a common center, which is God, and will come back after completing the circuit to the center from which we started. (5:271)

Vedanta knows no sin. There are mistakes but no sin; and in the long run everything is going to be all right. No Satan—none of this nonsense. Vedanta believes in only one sin, only one in the world, and it is this: the moment you think you are a sinner or anybody is a sinner, that is sin. From that follows every other mistake or what is usually called sin. There have been many mistakes in our lives. But we are going on. Glory be unto us that we have made mistakes! Take a long look at your past life. If your present condition is good, it has been caused by all the past mistakes as well as successes. Glory be unto success! Glory be unto mistakes! Do not look back upon what has been done. Go ahead! (8:126–27)

10

THE COUNSEL OF STRENGTH

Adjuncts of Fearlessness

If there is one word that you find coming out like a bomb from the Upanishads, bursting like a bomb-shell upon masses of ignorance, it is the word "fearlessness." And the only religion that ought to be taught is the religion of fearlessness. Either in this world or in the world of religion, it is true that fear is the sure cause of degradation and sin. It is fear that brings misery, fear that brings death, fear that breeds evil. (3:160)

Fill the brain with high thoughts, highest ideals, place them day and night before you, and out of that will come great work. Talk not about impurity, but say that we are pure. We have hypnotized ourselves into this thought that we are little, that we are born, and that we are going to die, and into a constant state of fear. (2:86)

We have to go back to philosophy to treat things as they are. We are suffering from our own karma. It is not the fault of God. What we do is our own fault, nothing else. Why should God be blamed? (6:53)

You have to realize truth and work it out for yourself according to your own nature. . . . All must struggle to be individuals— strong, standing on your own feet, thinking your own thoughts, realizing your own Self. No use swallowing doctrines others pass on—standing up together like soldiers in jail, sitting down together, all eating the same food, all nodding their heads at the same time. Variation is the sign of life. Sameness is the sign of death. (6:65)

For centuries people have been taught theories of degradation. They have been told that they are nothing. The masses have been told all over the world that they are not human beings. They have been so frightened for centuries, till they have nearly become animals. Never were they allowed to hear of the Atman. Let them hear of the Atman—that even the lowest of the low have the Atman within, which never dies and never is born—of Him whom the sword cannot pierce, nor the fire burn, nor the air dry—immortal, without beginning or end, the all-pure, omnipotent, and omnipresent Atman! (3:224)

The secret of life is not enjoyment, but education through experience. But, alas, we are called off the moment we begin really to learn. That seems to be a potent argument for a future existence. (5:150)

Whose meditation is real and effective? Who can really resign himself to the will of God? Who can utter with power irresistible, like that of a thunderbolt, the name of the Lord? It is he . . . whose mind has been purified by work. . . .
Every individual is a center for the manifestation of a certain force. This force has been stored up as the resultant of our previous works, and each one of us is born with this force at his back. So long as this force has not worked itself out, who can possibly remain quiet and give up work? Until then, he will have to enjoy or suffer according to the fruition of his good or bad work and will be irresistibly impelled to work. Since enjoyment and work cannot be given up till then, is it not better to do good rather than bad works—to enjoy happiness rather than suffer misery? (5:449–50)

No one knew why it would be good to love other beings as ourselves. And the reason why is there—in the idea of the Impersonal God; you understand it when you learn that the whole world is one—the oneness of the universe—the solidarity of all life—that in hurting anyone I am hurting myself, in loving anyone I am loving myself. Hence we understand why it is that we ought not to hurt others. (3:129–30)

As long as we believe ourselves to be even the least different from God, fear remains with us; but when we know ourselves to be the One, fear goes; of what can we be afraid? (8:10)

Those who are always downhearted and dispirited in this life can do no work; from life to life they come and go wailing and moaning. "The earth is enjoyed by heroes"—this is the unfailing truth. Be a hero. Always say, "I have no fear." Tell this to every-body—"Have no fear." Fear is death, fear is sin, fear is hell, fear is unrighteousness, fear is wrong life. All the negative thoughts and ideas that are in this world have proceeded from this evil spirit of fear. (7:136)

Stand Up and Be Strong

Stand up, be bold, be strong. Take the whole responsibility on your own shoulders, and know that you are the creator of your own destiny. All the strength and succor you want is within yourselves. Therefore, make your own future. (2:225)

If there is no strength in body and mind, the Atman cannot be realized. First you have to build the body by good nutritious food—then only will the mind be strong. The mind is but the subtle part of the body. You must retain great strength in your mind and words. "I am low, I am low"—repeating these ideas in the mind, man belittles and degrades himself. (7:135)

The greatest sin is to think yourself weak. No one is greater: realize you are Brahman. Nothing has power except what you give it. We are beyond the sun, the stars, the universe. Teach the

Godhood of man. Deny evil, create none. Stand up and say, I am the master, the master of all. We forge the chain, and we alone can break it. (7:54)

The sign of vigor, the sign of life, the sign of hope, the sign of health, the sign of everything that is good, is strength. As long as the body lives, there must be strength in the body, strength in the mind, in the hand. (6:62)

One who leans on somebody cannot serve the God of Truth. (5:72)

There is only one sin. That is weakness. . . . The only saint is that soul that never weakens, faces everything, and determines to die game.

Stand up and die game! . . . Do not add one lunacy to another. Do not add your weakness to the evil that is going to come. That is all I have to say to the world. Be strong! . . . You talk of ghosts and devils. We are the living devils. The sign of life is strength and growth. The sign of death is weakness. Whatever is weak, avoid! It is death. If it is strength, go down into hell and get hold of it! There is salvation only for the brave. "None but the brave deserves the fair." None but the bravest deserves salvation. Whose hell? Whose torture? Whose sin? Whose weakness? Whose death? Whose disease?

You believe in God. If you do, believe in the real God. "Thou art the man, Thou the woman, Thou the young man walking in the strength of youth. . . . Thou the old man tottering with his stick." Thou art weakness. Thou art fear. Thou art heaven, and Thou art hell. Thou art the serpent that would sting. Come Thou as fear! Come Thou as death! Come Thou as misery! . . . All weakness, all bondage is imagination. Speak one word to it, it must vanish. Do not weaken! There is no other way out. . . . Stand up and be strong! (1:479)

Freedom is never to be reached by the weak. Throw away all weakness. Tell your body that it is strong, tell your mind that it is strong, and have unbounded faith and hope in yourself. (1:146)

You know, there are bullock carts in India. Usually two bulls are harnessed to a cart, and sometimes a sheaf of straw is dangled at the tip of the pole, a little in front of the animals but beyond their reach. The bulls try continually to feed upon the straw, but never succeed. This is exactly how we are helped! We think we are going to get security, strength, wisdom, happiness from the outside. We always hope but never realize our hope. Never does any help come from the outside.

There is no help for man. None ever was, none is, and none will be. Why should there be? Are you not men and women? Are the lords of the earth to be helped by others? Are you not ashamed? You will be helped when you are reduced to dust. But you are spirit. Pull yourself out of difficulties by yourself! Save yourself by yourself! There is none to help you—never was. To think that there is, is sweet delusion. It comes to no good. (8:131–32)

Strength is the medicine for the world's disease. Strength is the medicine which the poor must have when tyrannized over by the rich. Strength is the medicine that the ignorant must have when oppressed by the learned; and it is the medicine that sinners must have when tyrannized over by other sinners; and nothing gives such strength as this idea of monism. Nothing makes us so moral as this idea of monism. Nothing makes us work so well at our best and highest as when all the responsibility is thrown upon ourselves. . . . If the whole responsibility is thrown upon our own shoulders, we shall be at our highest and best; and when we have nobody to grope toward, no devil to lay our blame upon, no Personal God to carry our burdens, when we are alone responsible, then we shall rise to our highest and best.

. . . This is the only way to reach the goal, to tell ourselves, and to tell everybody else, that we are divine. And as we go on repeating this, strength comes. He who falters at first will get stronger and stronger, and the voice will increase in volume until the truth takes possession of our hearts, and courses through our veins, and permeates our bodies. Delusion will vanish as the light becomes more and more effulgent, load after load of ignorance will vanish, and then will come a time when all else has disappeared and the sun alone shines. (2:201–2)

Why are people so afraid? The answer is that they have made themselves helpless and dependent on others. We are so lazy, we do not want to do anything for ourselves. We want a Personal God, a savior or a prophet to do everything for us. (8:131)

It is the cheerful mind that is persevering. It is the strong mind that hews its way through a thousand difficulties. And this, the hardest task of all, the cutting of our way out of the net of maya, is the work reserved only for giant wills. (3:69)

The karma yogi is the man who understands that the highest ideal is nonresistance, and who also knows that this nonresistance is the highest manifestation of power in actual possession, and also what is called the resisting of evil is but a step on the way toward the manifestation of this highest power, namely, nonresistance. Before reaching this highest ideal, man's duty is to resist evil; let him work, let him fight, let him strike straight from the shoulder. Then only, when he has gained the power to resist, will nonresistance be a virtue. (1:39)

Making Our Way

Don't look back—forward, infinite energy, infinite enthusiasm, infinite daring, and infinite patience—then alone can great deeds be accomplished. (8:353)

No great idea can have a place in the heart unless one steps out of his little corner. (6:331)

I fervently wish no misery ever came near anyone; yet it is that alone that gives us an insight into the depths of our lives, does it not? In our moments of anguish, gates barred forever seem to open and let in many a flood of light. (8:466)

Great work requires great and persistent effort for a long time. . . . Character has to be established through a thousand stumbles. (8:383)

Worship the Terrible! Worship Death! All else is vain. All struggle is vain. That is the last lesson. Yet this is not the coward's love of death, not the love of the weak or the suicide. It is the welcome of the strong man who has sounded everything to its depths and *knows* that there is no alternative. (8:266)

Blows are what awaken us and help to break the dream. They show us the insufficiency of this world and make us long to escape, to have freedom. (7:79)

This I have seen in life—he who is overcautious about himself falls into dangers at every step; he who is afraid of losing honor and respect, gets only disgrace; he who is always afraid of loss always loses. (8:433)

This life is a hard fact; work your way through it boldly, though it may be adamantine; no matter, the soul is stronger. It lays no responsibility on little gods; for you are the makers of your own fortunes. You make yourselves suffer, you make good and evil, and it is you who put your hands before your eyes and say it is dark. Take your hands away and see the light; you are effulgent, you are perfect already, from the very beginning. (2:182)

Have Faith in Yourself

The greatest religion is to be true to your own nature. Have faith in yourselves! (1:483)

Our first duty is not to hate ourselves, because to advance we must have faith in ourselves first and then in God. He who has no faith in himself can never have faith in God. (1:38)

Let people say whatever they like, stick to your own convictions, and rest assured, the world will be at your feet. They say, "Have faith in this fellow or that fellow," but I say, "Have faith in yourself first," that's the way. Have faith in yourself—all power is in you—be conscious and bring it out. Say, "I can do everything." (6:274)

Yes, if to know the secrets of the Atman, to liberate your soul, to reach the true solution of the mystery of birth and death, you have to go to the very jaws of death and realize the truth thereby, well, go there with an undaunted heart. It is fear alone that is death. You have to go beyond all fear. So from this day be fearless. (6:472–73)

There is no help for you outside of yourself; you are the creator of the universe. Like the silkworm you have built a cocoon around yourself. Who will save you? Burst your own cocoon and come out as the beautiful butterfly, as the free soul. Then alone you will see Truth. (3:26)

Struggle, struggle, was my motto for the last ten years. Struggle, still say I. When it was all dark, I used to say, struggle; when light is breaking in, I still say, struggle. (4:367)

Wait, money does not pay, nor name; fame does not pay, nor learning. It is love that pays; it is character that cleaves its way through adamantine walls of difficulties. (4:367)

Be independent, learn to form independent judgments. (6:265)

What is the true meaning of the assertion that we should depend on ourselves? Here self means the eternal Self. But even dependence on the noneternal self may lead gradually to the right goal, as the individual self is really the eternal Self under delusion. (5:314)

To believe blindly is to degenerate the human soul. Be an atheist if you want, but do not believe in anything unquestioningly. (4:216)

If any one of you believes what I teach, I will be sorry. I will only be too glad if I can excite in you the power of thinking for yourselves. (6:64)

Be free; hope for nothing from anyone. I am sure if you look back upon your lives you will find that you were always vainly trying to get help from others which never came. All the help that has come was from within yourselves. (2:324)

Buddha's idea is that there is no God, only man himself. He repudiated the mentality which underlies the prevalent ideas of God. He found it made men weak and superstitious. If you pray to God to give you everything, who is it, then, that goes out and works? God comes to those who work hard. God helps them that help themselves. An opposite idea of God weakens our nerves, softens our muscles, makes us dependent. Everything independent is happy; everything dependent is miserable. Man has infinite power within himself, and he can realize it—he can realize himself as the one infinite Self. It can be done; but you do not believe it. You pray to God and keep your powder dry all the time. (8:101–2)

11

WITHOUT THOUGHT OF SELF

The Law of Life

All expansion is life, all contraction is death. All love is expansion, all selfishness is contraction. Love is therefore the only law of life. He who loves lives, he who is selfish is dying. Therefore love for love's sake, because it is the only law of life, just as you breathe to live. (6:320)

Are you sincere? unselfish even unto death? and loving? Then fear not, not even death. (5:43)

It is unswerving love and perfect unselfishness that conquer everything. We Vedantists in every difficulty ought to ask the subjective question, "Why do I see that?" "Why can I not conquer this with love?" (8:383)

There are two things which guide the conduct of men: might and mercy. The exercise of might is invariably the exercise of selfishness. All men and women try to make the most of whatever power or advantage they have. Mercy is heaven itself; to be good, we have all to be merciful. Even justice and right should stand on mercy. (1:59)

The moment you isolate yourself, everything hurts you. The moment you expand and feel for others, you gain help. The selfish man is the most miserable in the world. The happiest is the man who is not at all selfish. (2:465)

How does the Vedanta explain individuality and ethics? The real individual is the Absolute; this personalization is through maya. It is only apparent; in reality it is always the Absolute. In reality there is one, but in maya it is appearing as many. In maya there is this variation. Yet even in this maya there is always the tendency to get back to the One, as expressed in all ethics and all morality of every nation, because it is the constitutional necessity of the soul. It is finding its oneness; and this struggle to find this oneness is what we call ethics and morality. Therefore we must always practice them. (5:309–10)

The Ego-Self in Light and Shadow

Whenever you think of yourself, you are bound to feel restless. (6:266)

It is that eternal love, unruffled equanimity under all circumstances, and perfect freedom from jealousy or animosity that will tell. That will tell, nothing else. (7:488)

Our best work is done, our greatest influence is exerted, when we are without thought of self. All great geniuses know this. Let us open ourselves to the one Divine Actor, and let Him act, and do nothing ourselves. (7:14)

It is selfishness that we must seek to eliminate. I find that whenever I have made a mistake in my life, it has always been because *self* entered into the calculation. Where self has not been involved, my judgment has gone straight to the mark. (8:265)

Every religion preaches that the essence of all morality is to do good to others. And why? Be unselfish. And why should I? Some God has said it? He is not for me. Some texts have declared it? Let them; that is nothing to me; let them all tell it. And if they do, what is it to me? Each one for himself, and somebody take the hindermost—that is all the morality in the world, at least with many. What is the reason that I should be moral? You cannot explain it except when you come to know the truth as given in the *Gita*: "He who sees everyone in himself, and himself in everyone, thus seeing the same God living in all, he, the sage, no more kills the Self by the self." Know through Advaita that whomsoever you hurt, you hurt yourself; they are all you. Whether you know it or not, through all hands you work, through all feet you move, you are the king enjoying in the palace, you are the beggar leading that miserable existence in the street; you are in the ignorant as well as in the learned, you are in the man who is weak, and you are in the strong; know this and be sympathetic. And that is why we must not hurt others. That is why I do not even care whether I have to starve, because there will be millions of mouths eating at the same time, and they are all mine. Therefore I should not care what becomes of me and mine, for the whole universe is mine, I am enjoying all the bliss at the same time; and who can kill me or the universe? Herein is morality. (3:425)

Love is always a manifestation of bliss. The least shadow of pain falling upon it is always a sign of physicality and selfishness. (8:276)

The adamantine wall that shuts us in is egoism; we refer everything to ourselves, thinking, "I do this, that, and the other." Get rid of this puny "I"; kill this diabolism in us; "Not I, but Thou"— say it, feel it, live it. Until we give up the world manufactured by the ego, never can we enter the kingdom of heaven. (7:15)

Truth can never come to us as long as we are selfish. We color everything with our own selves. Things come to us as they are. Not that they are hidden, not at all! *We* hide them. We have the brush. A thing comes, and we do not like it, and we brush a little and then look at it. . . . We do not want to know. We paint everything with ourselves. In all action the motive power is selfishness. Everything is hidden by ourselves. We are like the caterpillar which takes the thread out of his own body and of that makes the cocoon, and behold, he is caught. By his own work he imprisons himself. That is what we are doing. The moment I say "me" the thread makes a turn. "I and mine," another turn. So it goes. (1:476–77)

Are you unselfish? That is the question. If you are, you will be perfect without reading a single religious book, without going into a single church or temple. (1:93)

It is one of the evils of your Western civilization that you are after intellectual education alone, and take no care of the heart. It only makes men ten times more selfish, and that will be your destruction. (1:412)

The Only Positive Power

Can any man deny that love, this "not I," this renunciation is the only positive power in the universe? (2:354)

If you desire wealth, and know at the same time that the whole world regards him who aims at wealth as a very wicked man, you, perhaps, will not dare to plunge into the struggle for wealth, yet your mind will be running day and night after money. This is hypocrisy and will serve no purpose. Plunge into the world, and then, after a time, when you have suffered and enjoyed all that is in it, will renunciation come; then will calmness come. So fulfill your desire for power and everything else, and after you have fulfilled the desire, will come the time when you will know that they are all very little things; but until you have fulfilled this desire, until you have passed through that activity, it is impossible for you to come to the state of calmness, serenity, and self-surrender. (1:40)

Renunciation is the background of all religious thought wherever it be, and you will always find that as this idea of renunciation lessens, the more will the senses creep into the field of religion, and spirituality will decrease in the same ratio. (4:183–84)

Wherever there is attachment, the clinging to the things of the world, you must know that it is all physical attraction between sets of particles of matter—something that attracts two bodies nearer and nearer all the time and, if they cannot get near enough, produces pain; but where there is *real* love, it does not rest on physical attachment at all. Such lovers may be a thousand miles away from one another, but their love will be all the same; it does not die, and will never produce any painful reaction. (1:58–59)

I Am Not a Shopkeeper

All the teachers of humanity are unselfish. Suppose Jesus of Nazareth was teaching, and a man came and told him, "What you teach is beautiful. I believe that it is the way to perfection, and I am ready to follow it; but I do not care to worship you as the only begotten Son of God." What would be the answer of Jesus of Nazareth? "Very well, brother, follow the ideal and advance in your own way. I do not care whether you give me the credit for the teaching or not. I am not a shopkeeper. I do not trade in religion. I only teach truth, and truth is nobody's property. Nobody can patent truth. Truth is God Himself." (4:150)

The watchword of all well-being, of all moral good is not "I" but "thou." Who cares whether there is a heaven or a hell, who cares if there is a soul or not, who cares if there is an unchangeable or not? Here is the world, and it is full of misery. Go out into it as Buddha did, and struggle to lessen it or die in the attempt. Forget yourselves; this is the first lesson to be learnt, whether you are a theist or an atheist, whether you are an agnostic or a Vedantist, a Christian or a Muslim. The one lesson obvious to all is the destruction of the little self and the building up of the Real Self. (2:353)

Pure love has no motive. It has nothing to gain. (6:90)

Does one feel happy to taste of a good thing all by oneself? One should share it with others. Granted that you attain personal liberation by means of the realization of Advaita, but what matters it to the world? You must liberate the whole universe before you leave this body. Then only will you be established in the eternal Truth. Has that bliss any match, my boy? You will be established in that bliss of the Infinite which is limitless like the skies. You will be struck dumb to find your presence everywhere in the world of soul and matter. You will feel the whole sentient and insentient world as your own Self. Then you can't help treating all with the same kindness as you show toward yourself. This is indeed practical Vedanta. Do you understand me? Brahman is one, but is at the same time appearing to us as many, on the relative plane. (7:163)

Can you reach the realization of such an idea in which all sense of self is completely lost? It is a very dizzy height on the pinnacle of the religion of love, and few in this world have ever climbed up to it; but until a man reaches that highest point of ever-ready and ever-willing self-sacrifice, he cannot become a perfect bhakta. (3:83)

Great men are those who build highways for others with their heart's blood. This has been taking place through eternity, that one builds a bridge by laying down his own body, and thousands of others cross the river through its help. (6:273–74)

Those that want to help mankind must take their own pleasure and pain, name and fame, and all sorts of interests, and make a bundle of them and throw them into the sea, and then come to the Lord. This is what all the Masters *said* and *did*. (6:302)

The position of the mother is the highest in the world, as it is the one place in which to learn and exercise the greatest unselfishness. (1:68)

As the Rose Gives Perfume

Give as the rose gives perfume, because it is its own nature, utterly unconscious of giving. (7:86)

At the present time there are men who give up the world to help their own salvation. Throw away everything, even your own salvation, and go and help others. (3:431)

Even the least work done for others awakens the power within; even thinking the least good of others gradually instills into the heart the strength of a lion. (5:382)

All outgoing energy following a selfish motive is frittered away; it will not cause power to return to you; but if restrained, it will result in development of power. This self-control will tend to produce a mighty will, a character which makes a Christ or a Buddha. (1:33)

Be perfectly resigned, perfectly unconcerned; then alone can you do any true work. No eyes can see the real forces, we can only see the results. Put out self, lose it, forget it; just let God work, it is His business. We have nothing to do but stand aside and let God work. The more we go away, the more God comes in. Get rid of the little "I," and let only the great "I" live. (7:14)

God is in every man, whether man knows it or not; your loving devotion is bound to call up the divinity in him. (5:148)

When you help a poor man, do not feel the least pride. That is worship for you, and not the cause of pride. (2:237)

It is better to wear out than to rust out—especially for the sake of at least doing good to others. (7:176)

If you live in a cave, your thoughts will permeate even through the rock walls, will go vibrating all over the world for hundreds of years, maybe, until they will fasten on to some brain and work out there. Such is the power of thought, of sincerity, and of purity of purpose. (3:227)

The power is with the silent ones, who only live and love and then withdraw their personality. They never say "me" and "mine"; they are only blessed in being instruments. (7:16)

12

THE JOURNEY

Love—The Prime Mover

When you see man as God, everything, even the tiger, will be welcome. Whatever comes to you is but the Lord, the Eternal, the Blessed One, appearing to us in various forms, as our father, and mother, and friend, and child–they are our own soul playing with us. (2:326)

What is it that attracts man to man, man to woman, woman to man, and animals to animals, drawing the whole universe, as it were, toward one center? It is what is called love. Its manifestation is from the lowest atom to the highest being: omnipotent, all-pervading, is this love. What manifests itself as attraction in the sentient and the insentient, in the particular and in the universal, is the love of God. It is the one motive power that is in the universe. Under the impetus of that love, Christ gives his life for humanity, Buddha even for an animal, the mother for the child, the husband for the wife. It is under the impetus of the same love that men are ready to give up their lives for their country. (2:50–51)

Then alone a man loves when he finds that the object of his love is not any low, little, mortal thing. Then alone a man loves when he finds that the object of his love is not a clod of earth, but it is the veritable God Himself. The wife will love the husband the more when she thinks that the husband is God Himself. The husband will love the wife the more when he knows that the wife is God Himself. That mother will love the children more who thinks that the children are God Himself. That man will love his greatest enemy who knows that that very enemy is God Himself. That man will love a holy man who knows that the holy man is God Himself, and that very man will also love the unholiest of men because he knows the background of that unholiest of men is even He, the Lord. (2:286)

God is held to be "All-Love." . . . There is no love outside of Himself; the love that is in the heart with which you love Him is even He Himself. In a similar way, whatever attractions or inclinations one feels drawn by, are all He Himself. The thief steals, the harlot sells her body to prostitution, the mother loves her child—in each of these too is He! (5:336)

The unity of all existence—you all have it already within yourselves. None was ever born without it. However you may deny it, it continually asserts itself. What is human love? It is more or less an affirmation of that unity: "I am one with thee, my wife, my child, my friend!" (8:137)

Love binds, love makes for that oneness. You become one, the mother with the child, families with the city, the whole world becomes one with the animals. For love is Existence, God Himself; and all this is the manifestation of that One Love, more or less expressed. (2:304)

When a man comes in physical contact with his wife, the circumstances she controls through what prayers and through what vows! For that which brings forth the child is the holiest symbol of God himself. It is the greatest prayer between man and wife, the prayer that is going to bring into the world another soul fraught with a tremendous power for good or for evil. Is it a joke? Is it a simple nervous satisfaction? Is it a brute enjoyment of the body? (8:61)

The soul foolishly thinks of manifesting the Infinite in finite matter, Intelligence through gross particles; but at last it finds out its error and tries to escape. This going-back is the beginning of religion, and its method, destruction of self, that is, love. Not love for wife or child or anybody else, but love for everything else except this little self. (8:384)

Freely Offering

Do you ask anything from your children in return for what you have given them? It is your duty to work for them, and there the matter ends. In whatever you do for a particular person, a city, or a state, assume the same attitude toward it as you have toward your children—expect nothing in return. If you can invariably take the position of a giver, in which everything given by you is a free offering to the world, without any thought of return, then will your work bring you no attachment. Attachment comes only where we expect a return. (1:59)

Look at the torture the mother bears in bringing up the baby. Does she enjoy it? Surely . . . she loves it better than anything else. Why? Because there is no selfishness. (6:149)

The mother stands by her child through everything. Wife and children may desert a man, but his mother never! Mother, again, is the impartial energy of the universe, because of the colorless love that asks not, desires not, cares not for the evil in her child, but loves him the more. (8:252)

Never say "mine." Whenever we say a thing is "mine," misery will immediately come. Do not even say "my child" in your mind. Possess the child, but do not say "mine." If you do, then will come the misery. (1:100)

Selfishness is the devil incarnate in every man. Every bit of self, bit by bit, is devil. Take off self by one side and God enters by the other. When the self is got rid of, only God remains. Light and darkness cannot remain together. Forgetting the little "I" is a sign of a healthy and pure mind. A healthy child forgets its body. (6:119)

With love there is no painful reaction; love only brings a reaction of bliss; if it does not, it is not love; it is mistaking something else for love. When you have succeeded in loving your husband, your wife, your children, the whole world, the universe, in such a manner that there is no reaction of pain or jealousy, no selfish feeling, then you are in a fit state to be unattached. (1:58)

Even in selfishness, that self will multiply, grow and grow. That one self, the one man, will become two selves when he gets married; several, when he gets children; and thus he grows until he feels the whole world as his Self, the whole universe as his Self. He expands into one mass of universal love, infinite love—the love that is God. (2:51)

To Teach a Child

We have a peculiar idea in India. Suppose I had a child; I should not teach him any religion, but the practice of concentrating his mind; and just one line of prayer—not prayer in your sense, but this: "I meditate on Him who is the Creator of the universe; may He enlighten my mind." Then, when old enough, he goes about hearing the different philosophies and teachings, till he finds that which seems the truth to him. (8:254)

How many things we see in our childhood which we think to be good, but which really are evil, and how many things seem to be evil which are good! How the ideas change! (2:420)

It is good to be born in a church, but it is bad to die there. It is good to born a child, but bad to remain a child. Churches, ceremonies, and symbols are good for children, but when the child is grown, he must burst the church or himself. We must not remain children forever. (1:325)

The child is ushered into the world not as something flashing from the hands of nature, as poets delight so much to depict, but he has the burden of an infinite past; for good or evil he comes to work out his own past deeds. That makes the differentiation. This is the law of karma. Each one of us is the maker of his own fate. (3:124–25)

We, by our past actions, conform ourselves to a certain birth in a certain body, and the only suitable material for that body comes from the parents who have made themselves fit to have that soul as their offspring. (2:222)

No man was ever born who could stop his body one moment from changing. "Body" is the name of a series of changes. "As in a river the masses of water are changing before you every moment, and new masses are coming, yet taking similar form, so is it with this body." Yet the body must be kept strong and healthy. It is the best instrument we have. (1:142)

You cannot make a plant grow in soil unsuited to it. A child teaches itself. But you can *help* it to go forward in its own way. What you can do is not of the positive nature, but of the negative. You can take away the obstacles, but knowledge comes out of its own nature. Loosen the soil a little, so that it may come out easily. Put a hedge round it; see that it is not killed by anything, and there your work stops. You cannot do anything else. The rest is a manifestation from *within* its own nature. So with the education of a child; a child educates itself. You come to hear me, and when you go home, compare what you have learnt, and you will find you have thought out the same thing; I have only given it expression. I can never teach you anything: you will have to teach yourself, but I can help you perhaps in giving expression to that thought. (4:55)

Negative thoughts weaken men. Do you not find that where parents are constantly taxing their sons to read and write, telling them they will never learn anything, and calling them fools and so forth, the latter do actually turn out to be so in many cases? If you speak kind words to children and encourage them, they are bound to improve in time. What holds good of children, also holds good of children in the region of higher thoughts. If you can give them positive ideas, people will grow up to be men and learn to stand on their own legs. In language and literature, in poetry and the arts, in everything we must point out not the mistakes that people are making in their thoughts and actions, but the way in which they will gradually be able to do these things better. (7:170–71)

Teach It with a Voice of Thunder

I do not believe at all that monistic ideas preached to the world would produce immorality and weakness. On the contrary, I have reason to believe that it is the only remedy there is. If this be the truth, why let people drink ditch water when the stream of life is flowing by? If this be the truth, that they are all pure, why not at this moment teach it to the whole world? Why not teach it with the voice of thunder to every man that is born, to saints and sinners, men, women, and children, to the man on the throne and to the man sweeping the streets? (2:199)

Men are taught from childhood that they are weak and sinners. Teach them that they are all glorious children of immortality, even those who are the weakest in manifestation. Let positive, strong, helpful thought enter into their brains from very childhood. (2:87)

Why then do you make cowards of yourselves and teach your children that the highest state of man is to be like a dog, and go crawling before this imaginary being, saying that you are weak and impure, and that you are everything vile in this universe? (3:412)

We hear, "Be good," and "Be good," and "Be good," taught all over the world. There is hardly a child, born in any country in the world, who has not been told, "Do not steal," "Do not tell a lie," but nobody tells the child how he can help doing them. Talking will not help him. Why should he not become a thief? We do not teach him how not to steal; we simply tell him, "Do not steal." Only when we teach him to control his mind do we really help him. (1:171)

Foolish parents teach their children to pray, "O Lord, Thou has created this sun for me and this moon for me," as if the Lord has had nothing else to do than to create everything for these babies. Do not teach your children such nonsense. (1:88)

All truth is eternal. Truth is nobody's property; no race, no individual can lay any exclusive claim to it. Truth is the nature of all souls. Who can lay any special claim to it? But it has to be made practical, to be made simple, for the highest truths are always simple, so that it may penetrate every pore of human society, and become the property of the highest intellects and the commonest minds, of the man, woman, and child at the same time. (2:358)

From my childhood everyone around me taught weakness; I have been told ever since I was born that I was a weak thing. It is very difficult for me now to realize my own strength, but by analysis and reasoning I gain knowledge of my own strength, I realize it. All the knowledge that we have in this world, where did it come from? It was within us. What knowledge is outside? None. Knowledge was not in matter; it was in man all the time. Nobody ever created knowledge; man brings it from within. (2:339)

I have no objection to dualism in many of its forms. I like most of them, but I have objections to every form of teaching which inculcates weakness. This is the one question I put to every man, woman, or child, when they are in physical, mental, or spiritual training. Are you strong? Do you feel strength?—for I know it is truth alone that gives strength. I know that truth alone gives life, and nothing but going toward reality will make us strong, and no one will reach truth until he be strong. (2:201)

This one and only God is the "knownest" of the known. He is the one thing we see everywhere. All know their own Self, all know, "I am," even animals. All we know is the projection of the Self. Teach this to the children, they can grasp it. Every religion has worshiped the Self, even though unconsciously, because there is nothing else. (7:93)

13

THE MODES OF MATTER
AND MOTION

Everything Moves in a Circle

There is no motion in a straight line. Everything moves in a
circle; a straight line, infinitely produced, becomes a circle. If that
is the case, there cannot be eternal degeneration for any soul. It
cannot be. Everything must complete the circle, and come back to
its source. (2:231)

Every force completes a circuit. The force we call man starts
from the Infinite God and must return to Him. (6:138)

This tendency you will find throughout modern thought; in one
word, what is meant by science is that the explanations of things
are in their own nature, and that no external beings or existences
are required to explain what is going on in the universe. The
chemist never requires demons, or ghosts, or anything of that sort,
to explain his phenomena. The physicist never requires any one of
these to explain the things he knows, nor does any other scientist.
And this is one of the features of science which I mean to apply to
religion. In this religions are found wanting and that is why they
are crumbling into pieces. Every science wants its explanations
from inside, from the very nature of things; and the religions are
not able to supply this. (1:371)

The external and internal natures are not two different things;
they are really one. Nature is the sum total of all phenomena.
"Nature" means all that is, all that moves. We make a tremendous

distinction between matter and mind; we think that the mind is entirely different from matter. Actually, they are but one nature, half of which is continually acting on the other half. Matter is pressing upon the mind in the form of various sensations. These sensations are nothing but force. The force from the outside evokes the force within. From the will to respond to or get away from the outer force, the inner force becomes what we call thought.

Both matter and mind are really nothing but forces; and if you analyze them far enough, you will find that at root they are one. The very fact that the external force can somehow evoke the internal force shows that somewhere they join each other—they must be continuous and, therefore, basically the same force. When you get to the root of things, they become simple and general. Since the same force appears in one form as matter and in another form as mind, there is no reason to think matter and mind are different. Mind is changed into matter, matter is changed into mind. Thought force becomes nerve force, muscular force; muscular and nerve force become thought force. Nature is all this force, whether expressed as matter or mind.

The difference between the subtlest mind and the grossest matter is only one of degree. Therefore the whole universe may be called either mind or matter, it does not matter which. You may call the mind refined matter, or the body concretized mind; it makes little difference by which name you call which. All the troubles arising from the conflict between materialism and spirituality are due to wrong thinking. Actually, there is no difference between the two. (8:245–46)

Take any one of these most material sciences, such as chemistry or physics, astronomy or biology—study it, push the study forward and forward, and the gross forms will begin to melt and become finer and finer, until they come to a point where you are bound to make a tremendous leap from these material things into the immaterial. The gross melts into the fine, physics into metaphysics, in every department of knowledge. (4:204)

Whichever way we turn in trying to understand things in their reality, if we analyze far enough, we find that at last we come to a peculiar state of things, seemingly a contradiction: something which our reason cannot grasp and yet is a fact. We take up something—we know it is finite; but as soon as we begin to analyze it, it leads us beyond our reason, and we never find an end to all its qualities, its possibilities, its powers, its relations. It has become infinite. Take even a common flower, that is finite enough; but who is there that can say he knows all about the flower? There is no possibility of anyone's getting to the end of the knowledge about that one flower. The flower has become infinite—the flower which was finite to begin with. . . .

What is true of the flower, of the grain of sand, of the physical world, and of every thought, is a hundredfold more true of ourselves. We are also in the same dilemma of existence, being finite and infinite at the same time. We are like waves in the ocean; the wave is the ocean and yet not the ocean. There is not any part of the wave of which you cannot say, "It is the ocean." The name "ocean" applies to the wave and equally to every other part of the ocean, and yet it is separate from the ocean. So in this infinite ocean of existence we are like wavelets. At the same time, when we want really to grasp ourselves, we cannot—we have become the infinite. (2:397–98)

If that creative energy which is working all around us, day and night, stops for a second, the whole thing falls to the ground. There never was a time when that energy did not work throughout the universe, but there is the law of cycles, pralaya. Our Sanskrit word for "creation," properly translated, should be *projection* and not *creation*. For the word "creation" in the English language has unhappily got that fearful, that most crude idea of something coming out of nothing, creation out of nonentity, nonexistence becoming existence, which, of course, I would not insult you by asking you to believe. Our word, therefore, is projection. The whole of this nature exists, it becomes finer, subsides; and then after a period of rest, as it were, the whole thing is again projected forward, and the same combination, the same evolution, the same manifestations appear and remain playing, as it were, for a certain time, only again to break into pieces, to become finer and finer, until the whole thing subsides, and again comes out. Thus it goes on backward and forward with a wavelike motion throughout eternity. Time, space, and causation are all within this nature. To say, therefore, that it had a beginning is utter nonsense. No question can occur as to its beginning or its end. Therefore wherever in our scriptures the words "beginning" and "end" are used, you must remember that it means the beginning and end of one particular cycle; no more than that. (3:122–23)

The seed comes out of the tree; it does not immediately become a tree, but has a period of inactivity, or rather, a period of very fine unmanifested action. The seed has to work for some time beneath the soil. It breaks into pieces, degenerates as it were, and regeneration comes out of that degeneration. In the beginning, the whole of this universe has to work likewise for a period in that minute form, unseen and unmanifested, which is called chaos, and out of that comes a new projection. (2:206–7)

Take this whole evolutionary series, from the protoplasm at one end to the perfect man at the other, and this whole series is one life. In the end we find the perfect man, so in the beginning it must have been the same. Therefore, the protoplasm was the involution of the highest intelligence. You may not see it, but that involved intelligence is what is uncoiling itself until it becomes manifested in the most perfect man. That can be mathematically demonstrated. If the law of conservation of energy is true, you cannot get anything out of a machine unless you put it in there first. (2:208–9)

The Wave and the Ocean

The wave is the same as the ocean certainly, and yet we know it is a wave, and as such different from the ocean. What makes this difference? The name and the form; that is, the idea in the mind and the form. Now, can we think of a wave-form as something separate from the ocean? Certainly not. It is always associated with the ocean idea. If the wave subsides, the form vanishes in a moment, and yet the form was not a delusion. So long as the wave existed the form was there, and you were bound to see the form. This is maya.

The whole of this universe, therefore, is, as it were, a peculiar form; the Absolute is that ocean while you and I, and suns and stars, and everything else are various waves of that ocean. And what makes the waves different? Only the form, and that form is time, space, and causation, all entirely dependent on the wave. As soon as the wave goes, they vanish. As soon as the individual gives up this maya, it vanishes for him and he becomes free. The whole struggle is to get rid of this clinging on to time, space, and causation, which are always obstacles in our way. (2:136)

If you want to have life, you have to die every moment for it. Life and death are only different expressions of the same thing looked at from different standpoints; they are the falling and the rising of the same wave, and the two form one whole. (1:112–13)

Everything exists through eternity, and will exist through eternity. Only the movement is in succeeding waves and hollows, going back to fine forms, and coming out into gross manifestations. This involution and evolution is going on throughout the whole of nature. (2:208)

Our bodies are simply little whirlpools in the ocean of matter. (2:466)

All the actions that we see in the world, all the movements in human society, all the works that we have around us, are simply the display of thought, the manifestation of the will of man. (1:30)

Certain men stand up and say they have a communication from God and they are the mouthpiece of God Almighty, and no one else has the right to have that communication. This, on the face of it, is unreasonable. If there is anything in the universe, it must be universal; there is not one movement here that is not universal, because the whole universe is governed by laws. It is systematic and harmonious all through. Therefore what is anywhere must be everywhere. Each atom in the universe is built on the same plan as the biggest sun and the stars. If one man was ever inspired, it is possible for each and every one of us to be inspired, and that is religion. (4:215)

Every evolution presupposes an involution. Nothing can be evolved which is not already there. (2:227)

To every one of us there must come a time when the whole universe will be found to have been a mere dream, when we shall find that the soul is infinitely better than its surroundings. In this struggle through what we call our environments, there will come a time when we shall find that these environments were almost zero in comparison with the power of the soul. It is only a question of time, and time is nothing in the Infinite. It is a drop in the ocean. We can afford to wait and be calm. (1:421)

Subtle Forces and Influences

You see what is happening all around us. The world is one of influence. Part of our energy is used up in the preservation of our own bodies. Beyond that, every particle of our energy is day and night being used in influencing others. Our bodies, our virtues, our intellect, and our spirituality, all these are continuously influencing others; and so, conversely, we are being influenced by them. This is going on all around us. (2:13)

We must always remember that matter is only an infinitesimal part of the phenomena of nature. The vast part of phenomena which we actually see is not matter. For instance, in every moment of our life what a great part is played by thought and feeling, compared with the material phenomena outside! How vast is this internal world with its tremendous activity! The sense-phenomena are very small compared with it. (2:159)

We always find the causes of the gross in the subtle. The chemist takes a solid lump of ore and analyzes it; he wants to find the subtler things out of which that gross is composed. So with our thought and our knowledge; the explanation of the grosser is in the finer. The effect is the gross and the cause is the subtle. This gross universe of ours, which we see, feel, and touch, has its cause and explanation behind in the thought. The cause and explanation of that is also further behind. So in this human body of ours, we first find the gross movements, the movements of the hands and lips; but where are the causes of these? The finer nerves, the movements of which we cannot perceive at all, so fine that we cannot see or touch or trace them in any way with our senses, and yet we know they are the cause of these grosser movements. These nerve movements, again, are caused by still finer movements, which we call thought; and that is caused by something finer still behind, which is the soul of man, the Self, the Atman. In order to understand ourselves we have first to make our perception fine. No microscope or instrument that was ever invented will make it possible for us to see the fine movements that are going on inside; we can never see them by any such means. So the yogi has a science that manufactures an instrument for the study of his own mind, and that instrument is in the mind. The mind attains to powers of finer perception which no instrument will ever be able to attain. (8:193)

Nothing is entirely physical, nor yet entirely metaphysical; one presupposes the other and explains the other. All theists agree that there is a background to this visible universe; they differ as to the nature or character of that background. Materialists say there is no background. (7:42–43)

What is the most evolved notion that man has of this universe? It is intelligence, the adjustment of part to part, the display of intelligence, of which the ancient design theory was an attempt at expression. The beginning was, therefore, intelligence. At the beginning that intelligence becomes involved, and in the end that intelligence gets evolved. The sum total of the intelligence displayed in the universe must, therefore, be the involved universal intelligence unfolding itself. This universal intelligence is what we call God. (2:209–10)

14

THE WEB OF GOD, SOUL, AND NATURE

○

The Real and the Relative

Real existence, real knowledge, and real love are eternally connected with one another, the three in one: where one of them is, the others also must be; they are the three aspects of the One without a second—the Existence-Knowledge-Bliss. When that existence become relative, we see it as the world; that knowledge becomes in its turn modified into the knowledge of the things of the world; and that bliss forms the foundation of all true love known to the heart of man. (1:58)

There is but One, seen by the ignorant as matter, by the wise as God. (8:429)

There is but one Infinite Being in the universe, and that Being appears as you and as I; but this appearance of divisions is after all a delusion. He has not been divided, but only appears to be divided. This apparent division is caused by looking at Him through the network of time, space, and causation. When I look at God through the network of time, space, and causation, I see Him as the material world. When I look at Him from a little higher plane, yet through the same network, I see Him as an animal, a little higher as a man, a little higher as a god, but yet He is the One Infinite Being of the universe, and that Being we are. I am That, and you are That. Not parts of It, but the whole of It. (3:8)

The One becomes many. When we see the One, any limitations reflected through maya disappear; but it is quite true that the manifold is not valueless. It is through the many that we reach the One. (6:51)

It is only when one does not see another, does not feel another, when it is all one—then alone fear ceases, then alone death vanishes, then alone samsara vanishes. Advaita teaches us, therefore, that man is individual in being universal, and not in being particular. You are immortal only when you are the whole. You are fearless and deathless only when you are the universe; and then that which you call the universe is the same as that you call God, the same that you call existence, the same that you call the whole. It is the one undivided Existence which is taken to be the manifold world which we see, as do others who are in the same state of mind as we. (3:417)

In Every Living Being

Where shall we go to find God if we cannot see Him in our own hearts and in every living being? "Thou art the man, Thou art the woman, Thou art the girl, and Thou art the boy. Thou art the old man tottering with a stick. Thou art the young man walking in the pride of his strength." Thou art all that exists, a wonderful living God who is the only fact in the universe. This seems to many to be a terrible contradiction to the traditional God who lives behind a veil somewhere and whom nobody ever sees. (2:320)

From the highest to the lowest and most wicked man, in the greatest of human beings and the lowest of crawling worms under our feet, is the soul, pure and perfect, infinite and ever-blessed. In the worm that soul is manifesting only an infinitesimal part of its power and purity, and in the greatest man it is manifesting most of it. The difference consists in the degree of manifestation, but not in the essence. Through all beings exists the same pure and perfect soul. (6:24–25)

What is real? That which never changes, the Self of man, the Self behind the universe. (2:410)

There is the same pure white light—an emission of the divine Being—in the center of each, but the glass being of different colors and thickness, the rays assume diverse aspects in the transmission. The equality and beauty of each central flame is the same, and the apparent inequality is only in the imperfection of the temporal instrument of its expression. As we rise higher and higher in the scale of being, the medium becomes more and more translucent. (4:191)

It is impossible to find God outside of ourselves. Our own souls contribute all the divinity that is outside of us. We are the greatest temple. The objectification is only a faint imitation of what we see within ourselves. (7:59)

Each soul is a star, and all stars are set in that infinite azure, that eternal sky, the Lord. There is the root, the reality, the real individuality of each and all. Religion began with the search after some of these stars that had passed beyond our horizon, and ended in finding them all in God, and ourselves in the same place. (5:69)

I have been asked many times, "Why do you laugh so much and make so many jokes?" I become serious sometimes—when I have stomachache! The Lord is all blissfulness. He is the reality behind all that exists, He is the goodness, the truth in everything. You are His incarnations. That is what is glorious. The nearer you are to Him, the less you will have occasions to cry or weep. The further we are from Him, the more will long faces come. The more we know of Him, the more misery vanishes. If one who lives in the Lord becomes miserable, what is the use of living in Him? What is the use of such a God? Throw Him overboard into the Pacific Ocean! We do not want Him! (8:134)

The whole universe is one existence. There cannot be anything else. Out of diversities we are all going toward this universal existence. Families into tribes, tribes into races, races into nations, nations into humanity—how many wills going to the One! It is all knowledge, all science—the realization of this unity. (8:138)

Sharpening the Focus

This world is "the evolution of nature and the manifestation of God." It is our interpretation of Brahman or the Absolute, seen through the veil of maya or appearance. The world is not zero, it has a certain reality; it only *appears* because Brahman *is*. (8:3–4)

And what is salvation? To live with God. Where? Anywhere. Here, this moment. One moment in infinite time is quite as good as any other moment. (3:537)

All souls are playing, some consciously, some unconsciously. Religion is learning to play consciously. (5:270)

We are all like this in the world. A legend tells how once Narada said to Krishna, "Lord, show me maya." A few days passed away, and Krishna asked Narada to make a trip with him toward a desert. After walking for several miles, Krishna said, "Narada, I am thirsty; can you fetch some water for me?" "I will go at once, sir, and get you water." So Narada went. At a little distance there was a village; he entered the village in search of water and knocked at a door, which was opened by a most beautiful young girl. At the sight of her he immediately forgot that his Master was waiting for water, perhaps dying for the want of it. He forgot everything and began to talk with the girl. All that day he did not return to his Master. The next day, he was again at the house, talking to the girl. That talk ripened into love; he asked the father for the daughter, and they were married and lived there and had children. Thus twelve years passed. His father-in-law died, he inherited his property. He lived, as he seemed to think, a very happy life with his wife and children, his fields and his cattle, and so forth. Then came a flood. One night the river rose until it overflowed its banks and flooded the whole village. Houses fell, men and animals were swept away and drowned, and everything was floating in the rush of the stream. Narada had to escape. With one hand he held his wife, and with the other two of his children; another child was on his shoulders, and he was trying to ford this tremendous flood. After a few steps he found the current was too strong, and the child on his shoulders fell and was borne away. A cry of despair came from Narada. In trying to save that child, he lost his grasp upon one of the others, and it also was lost. At last his wife, whom he clasped with all his might, was torn away by the current, and he was thrown on the bank, weeping and wailing in bitter lamentation. Behind him there came a gentle voice, "My child, where is the water? You went to fetch a pitcher of water, and I am waiting for you; you have been gone for quite half an hour." "Half an hour!" Narada exclaimed. Twelve whole years had passed through his mind, and all these scenes had happened in half an hour! And this is maya. (2:120–21)

As much of you as my mind can grasp is what I know to be you and nothing more. In the same way, I am reading the Absolute, the Impersonal and see Him as Personal. As long as we have body and mind, we always see this triune being: God, nature, and soul. There must always be the three in one, inseparable. . . . There is nature. There are human souls. There is again That in which nature and the human souls are contained. (6:52)

The Book of Mind and Heart

The book one must read to learn chemistry is the book of nature. The book from which to learn religion is your own mind and heart. (6:81)

Knowledge of the Absolute depends upon no book, nor upon anything; it is absolute in itself. No amount of study will give this knowledge; it is not theory, it is realization. Cleanse the dust from the mirror, purify your own mind, and in a flash you know that you are Brahman. (7:34)

The world is neither true or untrue, it is a shadow of truth. (8:30)

The reality of everything is the same Infinite. This is not idealism; it is not that the world does not exist. It has a relative existence, and fulfills all its requirements. But it has no independent existence. It exists because of the Absolute Reality beyond time, space, and causation. (2:32–33)

The highest demonstration of reasoning that we have in any branch of knowledge can only make a fact probable, and nothing further. The most demonstrable facts of physical science are only probabilities, not facts yet. Facts are only in the senses. Facts have to be perceived, and we have to perceive religion to demonstrate it to ourselves. We have to sense God to be convinced that there is a God. We must sense the facts of religion to know that they are facts. Nothing else, and no amount of reasoning, but our own perception can make these things real to us, can make my belief firm as a rock. (4:167)

He has hidden himself inside the atom, this Ancient One who resides in the inmost recess of every human heart. The sages realized Him through the power of introspection, and got beyond both joy and misery. (2:165)

The Reality in Nature Is Spirit

The reality in nature is spirit. Reality itself—the light of the spirit—moves and speaks and does everything. It is the energy and soul and life of the spirit that is being worked upon in different ways by matter. . . . The spirit is the cause of all our thoughts and body-action and everything, but it is untouched by good or evil, pleasure or pain, heat or cold, and all the dualism of nature, although it lends its light to everything. (1:471)

Nature is like the chain of the Ferris wheel, endless and infinite, and these little carriages are the bodies or forms in which fresh batches of souls are riding, going up higher and higher until they become perfect and come out of the wheel. But the wheel goes on. (2:230)

Nature outside cannot give us any answer as to the existence of the soul, the existence of God, the eternal life, the goal of man, and all that. This mind is continually changing, always in a state of flux; it is finite, it is broken into pieces. How can nature tell of the Infinite, the Unchangeable, the Unbroken, the Indivisible, the Eternal? (3:252)

The Sanskrit word for creation is *srishti*, projection. What is meant by "God created things out of nothing"? The universe is projected out of God. He becomes the universe, and it all returns to Him, and again it proceeds forth, and again returns. Through all eternity it will go on in that way. (4:48)

If man's life is immortal, so also is the animal's. The difference is only in degree and not in kind. The amoeba and I are the same, the difference is only in degree; and from the standpoint of the highest life, all these differences vanish. A man may see a great deal of difference between grass and a little tree, but if you mount very high, the grass and the biggest tree will appear much the same. So, from the standpoint of the highest ideal, the lowest animal and the highest man are the same. If you believe there is a God, the animals and the highest creatures must be the same. (2:297)

Nature's task is done, this unselfish task which our sweet nurse, nature, had imposed upon herself. She gently took the self-forgetting soul by the hand, as it were, and showed him all the experiences in the universe, all manifestations, bringing him higher and higher through various bodies, till his lost glory came back, and he remembered his own nature. Then the kind mother went back the same way she came, for others who also have lost their way in the trackless desert of life. And thus is she working, without beginning and without end. And thus through pleasure and pain, through good and evil, the infinite river of souls is flowing into the ocean of perfection, of self-realization. (1:304)

The Absolute, to become nature, must be limited by time, space, and causation. (4:242)

Principles, Not Persons

There are these eternal principles which stand upon their own foundations without depending on any reasoning even, much less on the authority of sages however great, of incarnations however brilliant they may have been. We may remark that as this is the unique position in India, our claim is that the Vedanta only can be the universal religion, that it is already the existing universal religion in the world, because it teaches principles and not persons. No religion built upon a person can be taken up as a type by all the races of mankind. (3:250)

The Impersonal God is a living God, a principle. The difference between personal and impersonal is this, that the personal is only a man, and the impersonal idea is that He is the angel, the man, the animal, and yet something more which we cannot see, because impersonality includes all personalities, is the sum total of everything in the universe, and infinitely more besides. (2:319)

That God for whom you have been searching all over the universe is all the time yourself—yourself not in the personal sense but in the Impersonal. The man we know now, the manifested, is personalized, but the reality of this is the Impersonal. To understand the personal we have to refer it to the Impersonal, the particular must be referred to the general, and that Impersonal is the Truth, the Self of man. (2:334)

Matter does not prove Spirit. What connection is there between the existence of God, Soul, or immortality, and the working of miracles? (5:54–55)

Only the few dare to realize the God within, to renounce heaven, and Personal God and all hope of reward. A firm will is needed to do this; to be even vacillating is a sign of tremendous weakness. Man always *is* perfect, or he never could become so; but he had to realize it. If man were bound by external causes, he could only be mortal. Immortality can only be true of the unconditioned. (8:14–15)

15

HOW IT IS DONE

Goals

The spirit is the goal, and not matter. Forms, images, bells, candles, books, churches, temples, and all holy symbols are very good, very helpful to the growing plant of spirituality, but thus far and no farther. In the vast majority of cases, we find that the plant does not grow. It is very good to be born in a church, but it is very bad to die in a church. It is very good to be born within the limits of certain forms that help the little plant of spirituality, but if a man dies within the bounds of these forms, it shows that he has not grown, that there has been no development of the soul. (2:39–40)

A great sage once told me that not one in twenty million in this world believe in God. I asked him why, and he told me, "Suppose there is a thief in this room, and he gets to know that there is a mass of gold in the next room, and only a very thin partition between the two rooms; what will be the condition of that thief?" I answered, "He will not be able to sleep at all; his brain will be actively thinking of some means of getting at the gold, and he will think of nothing else." Then he replied, "Do you believe that a man could believe in God and not go mad to get him? If a man sincerely believes that there is that immense, infinite mine of Bliss, and that It can be reached, would not that man go mad in his struggle to reach it?" Strong faith in God and the consequent eagerness to reach Him constitute shraddha. (1:407)

That is the one great first step—the real desire for the ideal. Everything comes easy after that. (5:252)

The aim, the end, the goal, of all this training is liberation of the soul. Absolute control of nature, and nothing short of it, must be the goal. We must be the masters and not the slaves of nature; neither body nor mind must be our master, nor must we forget that the body is mine, and not I the body's. (1:140)

The success sometimes may come immediately, but we must be ready to wait patiently even for what may look like an infinite length of time. The student who sets out with such a spirit of perseverance will surely find success and realization at last. (3:48)

Meditate! The greatest thing is meditation. It is the nearest approach to spiritual life—the mind meditating. It is the one moment in our daily life that we are not all material—the Soul thinking of Itself, free from all matter—this marvelous touch of the Soul! (5:253)

There is a proverb in our language—"If I want to be a hunter, I'll hunt the rhinoceros; if I want to be a robber, I'll rob the king's treasury." What is the use of robbing beggars or hunting ants? So if you want to love, love God. (4:20)

If you can get absolutely still for just one moment, you have reached the goal. (6:96)

What is the ideal of the lover who has quite passed beyond the idea of selfishness, of bartering and bargaining, and who knows no fear? Even to the great God such a man will say, "I will give You my all, and I do not want anything from You; indeed there is nothing that I can call my own." (3:91)

Nonattachment is the basis of all the yogas. The man who gives up living in houses, wearing fine clothes, and eating good food, and goes into the desert, still may be a most attached person. His only possession, his own body, may become everything to him; and as he lives he will be simply struggling for the sake of his body.

Nonattachment does not mean anything that we may do in relation to our external body, it is all in the mind. The binding link of "I and mine" is in the mind. If we have not this link with the body and with the things of the senses, we are nonattached, wherever and whatever we may be. (1:101)

Here are the two ways of giving up all attachment. The one is for those who do not believe in God, or in any outside help. They are left to their own devices; they have simply to work with their own will, with the powers of their mind and discrimination, saying, "I must be nonattached." For those who believe in God there is another way, which is much less difficult. They give up the fruits of work unto the Lord; they work and are never attached to the results. Whatever they see, feel, hear, or do, is for Him. For whatever good work we may do, let us not claim any praise or benefit. It is the Lord's; give up the fruits unto Him. (1:102)

Nothing Is Done in a Day

Nothing is done in a day. Religion cannot be swallowed in the form of a pill. It requires hard and constant practice. The mind can be conquered only by slow and steady practice. (1:407)

Religion is a long, slow process. We are all of us babies here; we may be old, and have studied all the books in the universe, but we are all spiritual babies. We have learnt the doctrines and dogmas, but realized nothing in our lives. (4:36)

Practice is absolutely necessary. You may sit down and listen to me by the hour every day, but if you do not practice, you will not get one step further. It all depends on practice. We never understand these things until we experience them. We will have to see and feel them for ourselves. Simply listening to explanations and theories will not do. (1:139)

The test of progress is the amount of renunciation that one has attained. Where you find the attraction for lust and wealth considerably diminished, to whatever creed he may belong, know that his inner spirit is awakening. The door of Self-realization has surely opened for him. On the contrary if you observe a thousand outward rules and quote a thousand scriptural texts, still, if it has not brought the spirit of renunciation in you, know that your life is in vain. Be earnest over this realization and set your heart on it. (7:211)

The Beginnings

The preaching of sermons by brooks and stones may be true as a poetical figure but no one can preach a single grain of truth until he has it in himself. To whom do the brooks preach sermons? To that human soul only whose lotus of life has already opened. When the heart has been opened, it can receive teaching from the brooks or the stones—it can get some religious teaching from all these; but the unopened heart will see nothing but brooks and rolling stones. (4:27)

Purity is absolutely the basic work, the bedrock upon which the whole bhakti-building rests. Cleansing the external body and discriminating about food are both easy, but without internal cleanliness and purity, these external observances are of no value whatsoever. In the list of qualities conducive to purity, as given by Ramanuja, there are enumerated: truthfulness, sincerity, doing good to others without any gain to one's self, not injuring others by thought, word, or deed, not coveting others' goods, not thinking vain thoughts, and not brooding over injuries received from another. (3:67)

The man whose heart never cherishes even the thought of injury to anyone, who rejoices at the prosperity of even his greatest enemy, that man is the bhakta, he is the yogi, he is the guru of all, even though he lives every day of his life on the flesh of swine. Therefore we must always remember that external practices have value only as helps to develop internal purity. It is better to have internal purity alone when minute attention to external observances is not practicable. (3:68)

The repetition of names, the rituals, the forms, and the symbols, all these various things are for the purification of the soul. The greatest purifier among all such things, a purifier without which no one can enter the regions of this higher devotion, is renunciation. This frightens many; yet, without it, there cannot be any spiritual growth. In all our yogas this renunciation is necessary. This is the stepping-stone and the real center and the real heart of all spiritual culture—renunciation. This is religion—renunciation. (3:70)

Overcoming Obstacles

Fly from evil and terror and misery, and they will follow you. Face them, and they will flee. (1:339)

Live in the midst of the battle of life. Anyone can keep calm in a cave or when asleep. Stand in the whirl and madness of action and reach the Center. If you have found the Center, you cannot be moved. (6:84)

Many become wholly preoccupied with the outward forms and observances merely and fail to direct their mind to thoughts of the Atman! If you remain day and night within the narrow groove of ordinances and prohibitions, how will there be any expression of the soul? The more one has advanced in the realization of the Atman, the less is he dependent on the observances of forms. (7:211)

Now in intellectual development we can get much help from books, but in spiritual development, almost nothing. In studying books, sometimes we are deluded into thinking that we are being spiritually helped; but if we analyze ourselves, we shall find that only our intellect has been helped, and not the spirit. That is the reason why almost every one of us can *speak* most wonderfully on spiritual subjects, but when the time of action comes, we find ourselves so woefully deficient. It is because books cannot give us that impulse from outside. To quicken the spirit, that impulse must come from another soul. (4:22)

Above all, if the pride of spirituality enters into you, woe unto you. It is the most awful bondage that ever existed. Neither can wealth nor any other bondage of the human heart bind the soul so much as this. (1:429)

Varieties of Spiritual Practice

It is good to be born in a temple, but woe unto the person who dies in a temple or church. Out of it! . . . It was a good beginning, but leave it! It was the childhood place . . . but let it be! . . . Go to God directly. No theories, no doctrines. Then alone will all doubts vanish. Then alone will all crookedness be made straight.

In the midst of the manifold, he who sees that One; in the midst of this infinite death, he who sees that one life; in the midst of the manifold, he who sees that which never changes in his own soul— unto him belongs eternal peace. (2:474)

The man who thinks that he is receiving response to his prayers does not know that the fulfillment comes from his own nature, that he has succeeded by the mental attitude of prayer in waking up a bit of this infinite power which is coiled up within himself. (1:165)

The world is full of the talk of love, but it is hard to love. Where is love? How do you know that there is love? The first test of love is that it knows no bargaining. So long as you see a man love another only to get something from him, you know that that is not love; it is shopkeeping. Wherever there is any question of buying and selling, it is not love. So, when a man prays to God, "Give me this, and give me that," it is not love. How can it be? I offer you a prayer, and you give me something in return; that is what it is, mere shopkeeping. (2:47)

Bhakti yoga is the science of higher love. It shows us how to direct it; it shows us how to control it, how to manage it, how to use it, how to give it a new aim, as it were, and from it obtain the highest and most glorious results, that is, how to make it lead us to spiritual blessedness. Bhakti yoga does not say, "Give up"; it only says, "Love; love the Highest!"—and everything low naturally falls off from him, the object of whose love is the Highest. (3:73–74)

The renunciation necessary for the attainment of bhakti is not obtained by killing anything, but just comes in as naturally as in the presence of an increasingly stronger light, the less intense ones become dimmer and dimmer until they vanish away completely. So this love of the pleasures of the senses and of the intellect is all made dim and thrown aside and cast into the shade by the love of God Himself. (3:72)

He who cries out with his whole heart, "O Lord, I want but Thee"—to him the Lord reveals Himself. (6:88)

A finite subject cannot love, nor a finite object be loved. When the object of the love of a man is dying every moment, and his mind also is constantly changing as he grows, what eternal love can you expect to find in the world? There cannot be any real love but in God: why then all these loves? These are mere stages. There is a power behind impelling us forward, we do not know where to seek for the real object, but this love is sending us forward in search of it. Again and again we find out our mistake. We grasp something, and find it slips through our fingers, and then we grasp something else. Thus on and on we go, till at last comes light; we come to God, the only One who loves. His love knows no change and is ever ready to take us in. (4:15–16)

Why should we expect anything in return for what we do? Be grateful to the man you help, think of him as God. Is it not a great be allowed to worship God by helping our fellow men?

That self-existent One is far removed from the organs. The organs or instruments see outward, but the self-existing One, the Self, is seen inward. You must remember the qualification that is required: the desire to know this Self by turning the eyes inward. All these beautiful things that we see in nature are very good, but that is not the way to see God. We must learn how to turn the eyes inward. (2:411)

Sit in a straight posture, and the first thing to do is to send a current of holy thought to all creation. Mentally repeat, "Let all beings be happy; let all beings be peaceful; let all beings be blissful." So do to the east, south, north, and west. The more you do that the better you will feel yourself. You will find at last that the easiest way to make ourselves healthy is to see that others are healthy, and the easiest way to make ourselves happy is to see that others are happy. (1:145–46)

This power of meditation separates ourselves from the body, and then the soul knows itself as it is—the unborn, the deathless, and birthless being. No more is there any misery, no more births upon this earth, no more evolution. (4:249)

Controlling the passions is the next thing to be attended to. To restrain the indriyas [organs] from going toward the objects of the senses, to control them and bring them under the guidance of the will, is the very central virtue in religious culture. Then comes the practice of self-restraint and self-denial. All the immense possibilities of divine realization in the soul cannot get actualized without struggle and without such practice on the part of the aspiring devotee. (3:66)

What is the good of that spiritual practice or realization which does not benefit others, does not conduce to the well-being of people sunk in ignorance and delusion, does not help in rescuing them from the clutches of lust and wealth? Do you think, as long as one jiva endures in bondage, you will have any liberation? So long as he is not liberated—it may take several lifetimes—you will have to be born to help him, to make him realize Brahman. Every jiva is part of yourself—which is the rationale of all work for others. As you desire the wholehearted good of your wife and children, knowing them to be your own, so when a like amount of love and attraction for every jiva will awaken in you, then I shall know that Brahman is awakening in you, not a moment before. (7:235–36)

The mind must be made to quiet down. It is rushing about. Just as I sit down to meditate, all the vilest subjects in the world come up. The whole thing is nauseating. Why should the mind think thoughts I do not want it to think? I am, as it were, a slave to the mind. No spiritual knowledge is possible so long as the mind is restless and out of control. The disciple has to learn to control the mind. (8:110)

Let the mind run on and do not restrain it; but keep watch on your mind as a witness watching its action. This mind is thus divided into two—the player and the witness. Now strengthen the witnessing part and do not waste time in restraining your wanderings. The mind must think; but slowly and gradually, as the witness does its part, the player will come more and more under control, until at last you cease to play or wander. (6:135)

Each temperament has its own way. But this is the general principle: get hold of the mind. The mind is like a lake, and every stone that drops into it raises waves. These waves do not let us see what we are. The full moon is reflected in the water of the lake, but the surface is so disturbed that we do not see the reflection clearly. Let it be calm. Do not let nature raise the wave. Keep quiet, and then after a little while she will give you up. Then we know what we are. (4:248)

The greatest aid to the practice of keeping God in memory is, perhaps, music. The Lord says to Narada, the great teacher of bhakti, "I do not live in heaven, nor do I live in the heart of the yogi, but where My devotees sing My praise, there am I." Music has such tremendous power over the human mind; it brings it to concentration in a moment. You will find the dull, ignorant, low, brutelike human beings, who never steady their mind for a moment at other times, when they hear attractive music, immediately become charmed and concentrated. Even the minds of animals, such as dogs, lions, cats, and serpents, become charmed with music. (4:9)

The path of bhakti or devotion to God is a slow process, but is easy of practice. In the path of yoga there are many obstacles; perhaps the mind runs after psychic powers and thus draws you away from attaining your real nature. Only the path of jnana is of quick fruition and the rationale of all other creeds; hence it is equally esteemed in all countries and all ages. But even in the path of discrimination there is the chance of the mind getting stuck in the interminable net of vain argumentation. Therefore along with it, meditation should be practiced. By means of discrimination and meditation, the goal of Brahman has to be reached. One is sure to reach the goal by practicing in this way. This, in my opinion, is the easy path ensuring quick success. (7:198)

We do not know anything. This sort of humility will open the door of our heart for spiritual truths. Truth will never come into our minds so long as there will remain the faintest shadow of ahamkara (egotism). All of you should try to root out this devil from your heart. Complete self-surrender is the only way to spiritual illumination. (5:258)

Through the power of love the senses become finer and higher. The perfect love is very rare in human relations, for human love is almost always interdependent and mutual. But God's love is a constant stream, nothing can hurt or disturb it. (6:144)

Certain Religious Facts

There are certain religious facts which, as in external science, have to be perceived, and upon them religion will be built. Of course, the extreme claim that you must believe every dogma of a religion is degrading to the human mind. The man who asks you to believe everything, degrades himself, and, if you believe, degrades you too. The sages of the world have only the right to tell us that they have analyzed their minds and have found these facts, and if we do the same we shall also believe, and not before. That is all that there is in religion. (2:163)

All knowledge must stand on perception of certain facts, and upon that we have to build our reasoning. But curiously enough, the vast majority of mankind think, especially at the present time, that no such perception is possible in religion, that religion can only be apprehended by vain arguments. Therefore we are told not to disturb the mind by vain arguments. Religion is a question of fact, not of talk. We have to analyze our own souls to find what is there. We have to understand it and to realize what is understood. That is religion. No amount of talk will make religion. So the question whether there is a God or not can never be proved by argument, for the arguments are as much on one side as on the other. But if there is a God, He is in our own hearts. (2:162–63)

It will not do merely to listen to great principles. You must apply them in the practical field, turn them into constant practice. What will be the good of cramming the high-sounding dicta of the scriptures? You have first to grasp the teachings of the scriptures, and then to work them out in practical life. Do you understand? This is called practical religion. (7:117)

I do not deprecate the existence of sects in the world. Would to God there were twenty million more, for the more there are, the greater field for selection there will be. What I do object to is trying to fit one religion to every case. Though all religions are essentially the same, they must have the varieties of form produced by dissimilar circumstances among different nations. We must each have our own individual religion, individual so far as the externals of it go. (1:325–26)

This is the new religion of this age—the synthesis of yoga, knowledge, devotion, and work—the propagation of knowledge and devotion to all, down to the very lowest, without distinction of age or sex. (7:496)

Some are afraid that if the full truth is given to all, it will hurt them. They should not be given the unqualified truth—so they say. But the world is not much better off by compromising truth. What worse can it be than it is already? Bring truth out! If it is real, it will do good. (8:96)

What does the Advaitist preach? He dethrones all the gods that ever existed or ever will exist in the universe, and places on that throne the Self of man, the Atman, higher than the sun and the moon, higher than the heavens, greater than this great universe itself. No books, no scriptures, no science can ever imagine the glory of the Self that appears as man, the most glorious God that ever was, the only God that ever existed, exists, or ever will exist. (2:250)

16

FLOWERS AND THUNDERBOLTS

What the world wants is character. The world is in need of those whose life is one burning love, selfless. That love will make every word tell like a thunderbolt. (7:501)

Despondency is not religion, whatever else it may be. (4:11)

There is no chance for the welfare of the world unless the condition of women is improved. (6:328)

Soft-brained men, weak-minded, chicken-hearted, cannot find the truth. One has to be free, and as broad as the sky. (8:104)

If the mother is pleased, and the father, God is pleased with the man. (1:43)

Only that is ours which we earn. No authority can save us, no beliefs. If there is a God, *all* can find Him. No one needs to be told it is warm; each one can discover it for himself. So it should be with God. He should be a fact in the consciousness of all men. (8:15)

Words are only a mode of mind acting on mind. (6:34)

Religion as a science, as a study, is the greatest and healthiest exercise that the human mind can have. (2:66)

Let us not depend upon the world for pleasure. (8:29)

If superstition enters, the brain is gone. (3:278)

Let people have all the mythology they want, with its beautiful inspirations; for you must always bear in mind that emotional natures do not care for abstract definitions of truth. (2:393)

No man is born to any religion; he has a religion in his own soul. (6:82)

The great task is to revive the whole man, as it were, in order to make him the complete master of himself. (2:35)

Superstition is a great enemy of man, but bigotry is worse. (1:15)

Come out into the broad light of day, come out from the little narrow paths, for how can the infinite soul rest content to live and die in small ruts? Come out into the universe of Light. Everything in the universe is yours, stretch out your arms and embrace it with love. If you ever felt you wanted to do that, you have felt God. (2:322–23)

The new cycle must see the masses living Vedanta, and this will have to come through women. (7:95)

This earth is higher than all the heavens; this is the greatest school in the universe. (5:94)

This is no world. It is God Himself. In delusion we call it world. (6:371)

When you are judging man and woman, judge them by the standard of their respective greatness. (2:26)

The first sign that you are becoming religious is that you are becoming cheerful. (1:264)

This is the great lesson that we are here to learn through myriads of births and heavens and hells—that there is nothing to be asked for, desired for, beyond one's Self. (8:504)

Karma is the eternal assertion of human freedom. If we can bring ourselves down by our karma, surely it is in our power to raise ourselves by it. (5:213–14)

First, believe in this world—that there is meaning behind everything. (1:441)

We have no right to make others selfish by our own unselfishness, have we? (6:417)

There cannot be friendship without equality. (3:318)

You cannot believe in God until you believe in yourself. (5:409)

Nature, body, and mind go to death, not we; we never go nor come. (7:70)

Today God is being abandoned by the world because He does not seem to be doing enough for the world. So they say, "Of what good is He?" Shall we look upon God as a mere municipal authority? (7:18)

We are always after Truth, but never want to get it. (1:439)

Everything must be sacrificed, if necessary, for that one sentiment, *universality*. (6:285)

My ideal can be put into a few words and that is to preach unto mankind their divinity, and how to make it manifest in every movement of life. (7:501)

I believe in reason and follow reason. (2:336)

I shall not rest till I root out this distinction of sex. Is there any sex-distinction in the Atman (Self)? Out with the differentiation between man and woman—all is Atman! Give up the identification with the body, and stand up! (6:272–73)

Woman has suffered for eons, and that has given her infinite patience and infinite perseverance. (7:95)

All is the Self or Brahman. The saint, the sinner, the lamb, the tiger, even the murderer, as far as they have any reality, can be nothing else, because there is nothing else. (8:12)

What do you gain in heaven? You become gods, drink nectar, and get rheumatism. There is less misery there than on earth, but also less truth. (8:107)

In a conflict between the heart and the brain follow your heart. (8:223)

Every action that helps a being manifest its divine nature more and more is *good,* every action that retards is *evil.* (6:319)

Please everybody without becoming a hypocrite or a coward. (5:97)

Tell the truth boldly, whether it hurts or not. Never pander to weakness. If truth is too much for intelligent people and sweeps them away, let them go; the sooner the better. (7:79)

Stand as a rock; you are indestructible. You are the Self, the God of the universe. (2:236)

Go on saying, "I am free." Never mind if the next moment delusion comes and says, "I am bound." Dehypnotize the whole thing. (1:501)

How do you know that a book teaches truth? Because you are truth and feel it. That is what the Vedanta says. What is the proof of the Christs and Buddhas of the world? That you and I feel them. (2:307)

Be free! A free body, a free mind, and a free soul! That is what I have felt all my life; I would rather be free doing evil freely than be doing good under bondage. (3:515–16)

Too much sentiment hurts work. "Hard as steel and soft as a flower" is the motto. (8:434)

Various religions, Bibles, Vedas, dogmas—all are just tubs for the little plant; but it must get out of the tub. (7:6–7)

Do something for your souls! Do wrong if you please, but do something! (6:66)

Enough of books and theories. It is the *life* that is the highest and only way to stir the hearts of the people; it carries the personal magnetism. (5:65)

Perfection does not come from belief or faith. Talk does not count for anything. Parrots can do that. Perfection comes through the disinterested performance of action. (4:137)

Impurity is a mere superimposition under which your real nature has become hidden. But the real *you* is already perfect, already strong. (3:159)

The idea of perfect womanhood is perfect independence. (8:198)

Everything exists already in the Self of all beings. He who asserts he is free, shall be free. He who says he is bound, bound shall he remain. To me, the thought of oneself as low and humble is a sin and ignorance. (6:311)

Once I was invited to a dinner. The hostess asked me to say grace. I said, "I will say grace to you, madam. My grace and thanks are to you." (8:132–33)

Man finds nothing in that which does not echo back the heartbeats of his special love in life. (4:322)

Truth is infinitely more weighty than untruth; so is goodness. If you possess these, they will make their way by sheer gravity. (5:65)

I am glad I have done something good and many things bad; glad I have done something right, and glad I have committed many errors, because every one of them has been a great lesson. (2:147)

The pure heart is the best mirror for the reflection of truth. . . . All truth in the universe will manifest in your heart, if you are sufficiently pure. (1:414)

I would a hundred times rather have a little heart and no brain, than be all brains and no heart. . . . He who has no heart and only brains dies of dryness. (2:145)

Ordinarily speaking, spiritual aspiration ought to be balanced through the intellect; otherwise it may degenerate into mere sentimentality. (7:22)

Holiness is the greatest power. Everything else quails before it. (6:89)

Excepting the infinite spirit, everything else is changing. There is the whirl of change. Permanence is nowhere except in yourself. There is the infinite joy, unchanging. Meditation is the gate that opens that to us. (4:249)

When you deal with roots and foundations, all real progress must be slow. (5:193)

How easily this world can be duped by humbugs and what a mass of fraud has gathered over the devoted head of poor humanity since the dawn of civilization. (7:489)

People come to me—thousands come every year—with this one question. Someone has told them that if they are chaste and pure they will be hurt physically. . . . How do these teachers know it? Have they been chaste? These unchaste, impure fools, lustful creatures, want to drag the whole world down. (1:520)

Individuality is my motto. (7:487)

Salvation means knowing the truth. We do not become anything; we are what we are. . . . It is a question of *knowledge*! You must *know* what you are, and it is done. (1:512)

I have never seen the man who is not at least my equal. (6:48)

Contradictions come from the same truth adapting itself to the varying circumstances of different natures. (1:18)

God is the infinite, impersonal being—ever existent, unchanging, immortal, fearless; and you are all His incarnations, His embodiments. This is the God of Vedanta, and His heaven is everywhere. In this heaven dwell all the Personal Gods there are—you yourselves. (8:134)

We should be brave to open our doors to receive all available light from outside. Let rays of light come in, in sharp-driving showers from the four quarters of the earth. (4:406)

We cannot *know* Brahman, but we *are* Brahman, the whole of It, not a piece. (8:21)

All knowledge that we have, either of the external or internal world, is obtained through only one method—by the concentration of the mind. (4:219)

It is my belief that religious thought is in man's very constitution, so much so that it is impossible for him to give up religion until he can give up his mind and body, until he can give up thought and life. (3:1)

Every step I take in the light is mine forever. (7:59)

Wherever there is any love, any sweetness in any human being, either in a saint or a sinner, either in an angel or a murderer, either in the body, mind, or the senses, it is He. (2:421)

We must approach religion with reverence and with love, and our heart will stand up and say, this is truth, and this is untruth. (1:415)

The only knowledge that is of any value is to know that all this is humbug. But few, very few, will ever now this. "Know the Atman alone, and give up all other vain words." This is the only knowledge we gain from all this knocking about the universe. (8:35)

Learning and wisdom are superfluities, the surface glitter merely, but it is the heart that is the seat of all power. It is not in the brain but in the heart that the Atman, possessed of knowledge, power, and activity, has its seat. (6:425)

Jnana teaches that the world should be renounced but not on that account abandoned. To live in the world and not to be of it is the true test of renunciation. (5:272)

We must have friendship for all; we must be merciful toward those that are in misery; when people are happy, we ought to be happy; and to the wicked we must be indifferent. These attitudes will make the mind peaceful. (1:222)

The power of purity—it is a definite power. (4:33)

One word of truth can never be lost; for ages it may be hidden under rubbish, but it will show itself sooner or later. Truth is indestructible, virtue is indestructible, purity is indestructible. (5:57)

It is feeling that is the life, the strength, the vitality, without which no amount of intellectual activity can reach God. (2:307)

Worship of society and popular opinion is idolatry. The soul has no sex, no country, no place, no time. (8:37)

The Lord is very merciful to him whom He sees struggling heart and soul for realization. But remain idle, without any struggle, and you will see that His grace will never come. (5:398)

If you talk all the best philosophies the world ever produced, but if you are a fool in your behavior, they do not count. (3:536)

Who makes us ignorant? We ourselves. We put our hands over our eyes and weep that it is dark. (2:356)

Astrology and all these mystical things are generally signs of a weak mind; therefore as soon as they are becoming prominent in our minds, we should see a physician, take good food, and rest. (8:184)

Anything that brings spiritual, mental, or physical weakness, touch it not with the toes of your feet. (8:185)

The whole secret of existence is to have no fear. Never fear what will become of you, depend on no one. Only the moment you reject all help are you free. (7:49)

The first test of true teaching must be that the teaching should not contradict reason. (2:390)

Women will work out their own destinies—much better, too, than men can ever do for them. All the mischief to women has come because men undertook to shape the destiny of women. (8:91)

In worshiping God we have always been worshiping our own hidden Self. The worst lie that you ever tell yourself is that you were born a sinner or a wicked man. (2:279)

Wherever you are, that is a point from which you can start to the center. (3:536)

Suggestions for Further Reading

Anyone interested in a more extensive reading list may write to the Vivekananda Foundation, P.O. Box 1351, Alameda, CA 94501, for a bibliography and a list of sources for books.

Books by Vivekananda

Jnana Yoga. Edited by Swami Nikhilananda. New York: Rama-krishna-Vivekananda Center, 1982. Paperback, 317 pp.

Karma Yoga and Bhakti Yoga. Edited by Swami Nikhilananda. New York: Ramakrishna-Vivekananda Center, 1982. Paperback, 316 pp.

Raja Yoga. Edited by Swami Nikhilananda. New York: Ramakrishna-Vivekananda Center, 1982. Paperback, 297 pp.

The Complete Works of Swami Vivekananda, 8 vols. Calcutta: Advaita Ashrama, 1984–87. Paperback.

Vivekananda: The Yogas and Other Works. Edited by Swami Nikhi-lananda. New York: Ramakrishna-Vivekananda Center, 1984. Hardcover, 1018 pp. Includes *Jnana Yoga, Raja Yoga, Bhakti Yoga, Karma Yoga,* and *Inspired Talks*; lectures, poems, and letters; a biographical sketch; and twenty-five photographs.

Vedanta Voice of Freedom. Edited by Swami Chetanananda. St. Louis, Mo.: Vedanta Society of St. Louis, 1990. Paperback, 328 pp. Fifteen photographs. This book is a rearrangement of Vivekan-anda's thought into twelve chapters that explain the basic concepts of Vedanta.

Books about Vivekananda

Burke, Marie Louise. *Swami Vivekananda in the West: New Discoveries.* 8 vols. Calcutta: Advaita Ashrama, 1983–87. Hardcover. A complete account of Vivekananda's two stays in the West (1893–97 and 1899–1900).

Dhar, Sailendranath. *A Comprehensive Biography of Swami Viveka-nanda.* 2 vols. Madras: Vivekananda Prakashan Kendra, 1975–76. Hardcover.

Eastern and Western Disciples. *The Life of Swami Vivekananda.* 2 vols. Calcutta: Advaita Ashrama, 1979–81. Hardcover.

Swami Nikhilananda. *Vivekananda: A Biography.* New York: Rama-krishna-Vivekananda Center, 1989. Paperback. 216 pp. A useful, compact study.

Reminiscences of Swami Vivekananda. Calcutta: Advaita Ashrama, 1983. Paperback. 429 pp. A collection of thirty-five first-hand recollections of Vivekananda by Eastern and Western admirers.

Rolland, Romain. *The Life of Vivekananda and the Universal Gospel.* Calcutta: Advaita Ashrama, 1988. Paperback. First published in 1930, this work offers many insights into Vivekananda's life and message.

Glossary

ABSOLUTE. In Sanskrit, *Brahman*, the unconditioned Reality behind creation; Universal Self.

ADVAITA. Lit., "not two, nondual"; in *Vedanta* philosophy, the teaching that the individual Soul, the Absolute, and the universe are one.

AHAMKARA. Lit., "I-maker; I-ness"; ego; the concept of individuality.

ATMAN. The Self; the substratum of the individual self, which according to Advaita is identical with *Brahman*.

BHAGAVAD-GITA. Lit., "Song of God"; part of the Indian epic *Mahabharata*; on the battlefield, the Lord *Krishna* instructs Arjuna, a warrior-prince, on the proper methods of fulfilling his duties.

BHAKTA. A person who seeks God through devotion (bhakti) to His personal aspect in the form of a specific deity.

BHAKTI YOGA. The path to God-realization through devotion.

BRAHMAN. The *Absolute*; the Supreme Spirit; the self-existent, Impersonal One without a second.

BUDDHA. Lit., "the enlightened one"; the term often refers to the historical Buddha (Shakyamuni Buddha, fl. c. sixth century B.C.E.), the founder of Buddhism.

BUDDHI. The intellect; the mind's faculty of reason and discrimination.

DHARMA-MEGHA. The cloud of virtue.

DISCRIMINATION. In Sanskrit, *viveka*; the act of distinguishing between the real (the unchanging *Absolute*) and the unreal (what is transient; the manifest creation).

DIVINE MOTHER. The Supreme Goddess; the primal energy of the universe; the source of the creation.

GITA. See *Bhagavad-Gita*.

GURU. A spiritual teacher.

IGNORANCE. Spiritual blindness; mistaking the unreal for the real; on a cosmic scale, *maya*.

IMPERSONAL GOD. The *Absolute*; *Brahman*; God without qualities.

INDRIYAS. Internal organs of perception.

JIVA. The embodied soul; the living being; the ordinary person.

JIVANMUKTA. One who is liberated while still in the body.

JNANA YOGA. The path of God-realization through knowledge and discrimination.

JNANI. One who seeks Self-knowledge, the ultimate Reality.

KARMA. Action; work; law of cause and effect in the moral world.

KARMA YOGA. The path of God-realization through selfless action.

KNOWLEDGE. Frequently used to denote knowledge of spiritual Truth, knowledge of the immutable Reality in all things, or jnana.

KRISHNA. An incarnation of God; portrayed in the *Bhagavad-Gita* as the spiritual teacher of Prince Arjuna.

MASTER. A spiritual teacher; a person who has had spiritual experience and who is genuinely able to instruct others in spiritual matters; Vivekananda referred to *Shri Ramakrishna* as his master.

MAYA. Principle of illusion; cosmic illusion resulting in the One appearing as many.

MONOISM Nondualism; *Advaita*.

MUKTI. Liberation from the bondage of illusion and ignorance.

NARADA. A great sage and lover of God.

NIRVANA. Freedom; extinction or "blowing out" of delusions.

NONATTACHMENT. Dispassion for the world; internal renunciation; Skt., *vairagya*; see *renunciation*.

PERSONAL GOD. God with attributes, with or without form; the Supreme Person.

PRALAYA. Lit., "dissolution," destruction of the universe; disappearance of the material universe at the end of the cycle of manifestation.

PURITY. Internal and external cleanliness; a prerequisite for control of the mind.

RAMANUJA. Founder of the Visishtadvaita (Qualified Nondualism) school of *Vedanta*; he taught that reality is the Absolute in which qualities inhere, and that the individual soul is part of *Brahman*.

RENUNCIATION. Spirit of detachment brought about by *discrimination*; external renunciation is signified by the taking of vows; internal renunciation by the practice of detachment alone.

RAJA YOGA. One of the four main *yogas*; stresses concentration and meditation as methods of attainment.

SAMADHI. Experience of supreme consciousness; a superconscious state in which ultimate Reality is realized.

SAMSKARAS. Tendencies of the mind resulting from actions in previous births.

SAMSARA. The phenomenal world; the round of birth and death.

SANSKRIT. Ancient language of India; language of the *Vedas* and *Upanishads*.

SAT-CHIT-ANANDA. Lit., "Existence-Knowledge-Bliss"; a name of *Brahman*.

SELF. Eternal Self, *Atman;* identical with the Universal Spirit or *Brahman*.

SOUL. *Atman*; the eternal self.

SOUL. The individual soul as distinguished from the eternal Self (*Atman*); the *jiva*.

SHRADDHA. Faith; positive frame of mind; attitude necessary to Self-knowledge and love of god.

SHRI RAMAKRISHNA. Nineteenth-century Bengali knower of God, worshiped as a divine incarnation; Vivekananda's teacher.

SRISHTI. Lit., "letting go, letting loose"; creation of the universe; evolution of the universe from its seed state.

SWAMI. Lit., "master"; respectful title of address for a Hindu monastic.

TAMAS. Darkness; inertia.

TAPASYA. Devout austerity.

UPANISHADS. Sanskrit texts containing the records of the realizations of the ancient sages; the philosophical portion of the *Vedas*.

VEDANTA. Lit., "end of the Vedas"; the philosophy of the *Upanishads*; one of the six orthodox systems of Indian philosophy, it holds that the ultimate reality is *Brahman-Atman*, and that knowledge of the identity of the soul with Brahman is the key to liberation.

VEDAS. The ancient scriptures of India; revealed knowledge.

YOGA. Any of the various methods of attaining to spiritual liberation: i.e., *karma yoga*, the path of action; *jnana yoga*, the path of knowledge or philosophy; *bhakti yoga*, devotion to God; *raja yoga*, control of the mind.

YOGI. A practitioner of *yoga*.

(*Continued on next page*)

The Vimalakirti Nirdesa Sutra. Translated & edited by Charles Luk. Foreword by Taizan Maizumi Roshi.

Vitality, Energy, Spirit: A Taoist Sourcebook. Translated & edited by Thomas Cleary.

Wen-tzu: Understanding the Mysteries, by Lao-tzu. Translated by Thomas Cleary.

Worldly Wisdom: Confucian Teachings of the Ming Dynasty. Translated & edited by J. C. Cleary.

Zen Dawn: Early Zen Texts from Tun Huang. Translated by J. C. Cleary.

Zen Essence: The Science of Freedom. Translated & edited by Thomas Cleary.

Zen Teachings of Lin Chi. Translated by Burton Watson.

Made in the USA
San Bernardino, CA
22 February 2013